CQI for EMS

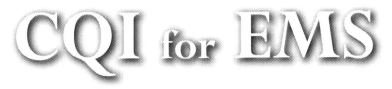

a practical manual
for QUICK results

Joseph Hayes III, NREMT-P
David Jaslow, MD, MPH, FAAEM

iUniverse, Inc.
Bloomington

CQI FOR EMS
A PRACTICAL MANUAL FOR QUICK RESULTS

iUniverse books may be ordered through booksellers or by contacting:

iUniverse
1663 Liberty Drive
Bloomington, IN 47403
www.iuniverse.com
1-800-Authors (1-800-288-4677)

ISBN: 978-1-4620-2618-0 (sc)
ISBN: 978-1-4620-2619-7 (ebk)

Printed in the United States of America

iUniverse rev. date: 07/23/2011

CONTENTS

Dedicated to all quality improvement coordinators

past, present, and future

who take on the glamorless, thankless,

yet most important job in EMS

ACKNOWLEDGMENTS

Scott Bahner, BS, NREMT-P

Lawrence Brilliant, MD

Barry Burton, DO, FACOEP, RN, EMT-P

Kimberly Dicken, EMT-B

Scott M. Henley, M.Ed., NREMT-P

Anne Klimke, MD, MS

Christine Landes, NREMT-P

Ken Lavelle, MD, FACEP, NREMT-P

Charles Pressler, EMT-P

Layne Shore, EMT-P

Christopher Sole, EMT-B

Samuel Wargny, EMT-P

FOREWORD

This book is based on similar continuous quality improvement programs conducted at two midsized, third service EMS agencies in Bucks County, Pennsylvania.

Thanks to the Bucks County Rescue Squad, located in Bristol, Pennsylvania, and Central Bucks Ambulance in Doylestown, a comparative study in quality improvement for EMS can be presented for the benefit of other EMS providers.

When most people think of EMS, their thoughts immediately turn to LA County Fire Department, New York City EMS, or systems in other big cities. But 90 percent of all EMS agencies in the United States are small to medium sized. Consequently, they face constraints in organization, financial resources, and personnel, which make developing and managing a quality improvement program a challenge.

Bucks County Rescue Squad and Central Bucks Ambulance cared enough about the quality of their patient care to take an objective look at what was going on at their agencies. They asked hard questions, made tough decisions, and broke with decades of tradition and precedent to do what had to be done to correct long-standing problems and deficiencies to dramatically improve the quality of their care.

Anatomy, physiology, and pathophysiology are all the same whether the patient is in Bucks County, Pennsylvania, or Bogalusa, Louisiana, and so are most quality of care issues. For the most part, we all have the same problems. The only question is whether you're aware you have these problems and whether you have a comprehensive process in place to resolve them or not.

To date, very few books have been written on the subject of quality improvement for EMS. Those which have been, have typically been written at the academic level, are too long winded and drawn out, too focused on theory, and too steeped in the history of quality control in industry. These books were simply not tailored or well suited for EMS. While most of those books make a good case for the need to improve patient care, they are typically presented too abstractly to be of much practical use. And so the decision was made to write a book on quality improvement specifically designed for EMS, a how-to book that presents specific actions and ideas that have been tried and proven with reproducible results at the two aforementioned EMS agencies. *CQI for EMS* can literally be read one day and put into effect the next, with the potential for quick results in just days or weeks. *CQI for EMS* is not designed to be the last word in quality improvement, it is just designed to help get you started.

Ken Lavelle, MD, FACEP, NREMT-P
Medical Director, Central Bucks Ambulance

10 Commandments
of
Quality EMS

1. EMS is not just a job, it is a profession.

2. Average, minimum, and mediocre are not good enough in EMS.

3. Always remember, your patients are trusting you with their lives.

4. Everyone gets to pick their primary care physician, but no one gets to pick their EMS provider.

5. Remember, the "S" in EMS stands for service.

6. You don't win points by guessing right in EMS. You win points by maintaining a high index of suspicion, finding problems that aren't so obvious, and always erring on the side of caution.

7. There are no excuses in EMS. You either get the job done or you don't.

8. In most cases, patients will be more appreciative of how you treat them than the treatments you give to them.

9. EMS is the first hour of medicine in the first thirty minutes.

10. Always treat your patients the way you'd want EMS to treat you or your family.

CHAPTER 1

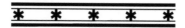

Quality in EMS: A History of Failure

Failure is not falling down, it's staying there.
—Benjamin Franklin

EMS is not industry: No book on the subject of quality improvement would be complete without mentioning W. Edward Deming and Malcolm Baldrige. So there you go—they've been mentioned.

Unlike other books written on quality improvement in EMS, we do not intend to waste your time on theory borrowed from industry and suggest you try to apply those abstracts to EMS. Rather, what we will attempt to do is keep this as short, sweet, and to the point as possible with some pertinent and usable background information. In the end, we hope to arm you with enough basic knowledge and tools to initiate a quality improvement program that will quickly and dramatically begin to improve your agency's quality of patient care, save lives, reduce risk, and make you, the quality improvement coordinator, look like a genius in the process.

The challenge of instilling quality in EMS has been around for as long as modern-day EMS. Any EMS veteran will recall initiatives such as Quality Assurance, Total Quality Management, Continuous Performance Improvement, and now, the latest catchphrase, Continuous Quality Improvement (CQI). It's like a tenement that catches fire and burns every few years; as soon as they rebuild it, they change the name in an attempt to erase the memory of the failure. So it has been with many quality programs in EMS.

Despite the lack of theory and history of quality in industry presented here, it might be useful to review the history of failed quality programs in EMS to give you some background and understanding of the scope of the problem.

Educational deficit: Let's start at the beginning, with the education deficit. Doctors complete four years of college, go on to four years of medical school, and then spend an additional three or four years in internship and residency. This is where they begin to practice medicine under the watchful eye of an experienced, senior physician. These mentors teach them the practical application of medicine, review their diagnoses, and sign off on their treatment—for three or four years, mind you. Nurses take two to four years of college and have their own clinical internship, where teaching nurses mentor them in a similar way as physicians. It's worth noting that despite all of their education and training, nurses are fairly restricted in their application of medicine; it's always under the direction of a doctor (with the exception of advanced practice nurses such as nurse practitioners).

Then you have the medics. For all intents and purposes, paramedics practice physician-level medicine, though much more limited and focused in scope. But compared to the educational requirements of a physician or nurse, most paramedics on the street today complete between twelve and eighteen months of training. Back when I became a medic in the 1980s, we were referred to as nine-month medical wonders . . . among other things, due to the fact that we learned all our emergency medicine in that very abbreviated amount of time.

After completing the paramedic course, a new medic typically does a preceptorship, which typically lasts from three to six months. This is where the new medic is mentored by a senior medic, who is typically a product of the same express line system of emergency medicine, after which the new medic is turned loose on society. Using myself as an example, I finished my nine months of medic school, completed a three-month preceptorship, and then spent the next twenty years repetitiously doing what little I was trained to do.

In twenty years, I received exactly five letters of inquiry from the quality assurance committee. Twenty years, thousands of patients, and just five questions asked. I'd like to think I was that good, and at the time, if you asked me, I probably would have told you I was. But in retrospect, knowing what I know today, I am much more humble.

Given the meager amount of medical training I received, it's hard to imagine that I didn't make all kinds of mistakes along the way. But if no one ever catches your mistakes and points them out to you, how would you ever know? You wouldn't, and I didn't. But with the exception of some high performance systems such as Medic One in San Francisco, Wake County EMS in North Carolina, and a handful of others, most systems continue to operate like this today.

Short of manning all ambulances with doctors, it's not possible to achieve the same educational standards for medics as physicians. But since the pathology, risks, and stakes are the same for the patient regardless of whether they're initially seen by a doc in the ER or medic in the field, common sense dictates that quality review and improvement are critical to trying to close the standard of care gap as much as possible. It would also seem to make sense that index of suspicion and caution should be increased, not decreased, in EMS from hospital standards.

Physician vs. medic standard of care: If I haven't already made my point, let me give you another example to emphasize the craziness. I've always tried to be a diligent paramedic who attempts to maintain a high index of suspicion and cast a wide net in hopes of catching all the critical (and potentially critical) patients. A couple of years ago, I arrived on the scene of a call for chest pain. The patient was a forty-five-year-old man who presented conscious and oriented and in no apparent distress. His vital signs were unremarkable. His only past medical history was gastric esophageal reflux disease (GERD). He described his discomfort as a burning sensation radiating up his chest into his neck. He had just finished a spicy dish at a local Mexican restaurant a couple hours before. There were no other associated complaints or symptoms. I quickly determined it was a likely exacerbation of his GERD, climbed into the front of the ambulance, and drove to the hospital; my EMT rode in the back with the patient. Who in EMS hasn't made such a clear-cut field diagnosis as this (and many others not so clear)?

We transported the patient and gave our report to the ER doc, who graciously accepted the patient without questioning my working diagnosis. He then turned to the nurse and ordered an IV, blood draw, and 12-lead EKG—all the things I could have done twenty minutes sooner but felt were unnecessary.

Being the inquisitive medic I am, I quickly discovered that standard hospital policy is any patient who comes to the ER by walk-in, ambulance, or double jointed jackass and who utters the words "chest pain" or "chest discomfort" is immediately ushered to an exam room, where despite any exclusionary criteria, they will receive all the aforementioned diagnostics. If the doctor (who if you will recall has a total twelve years of medical training to a paramedic's average of twelve months) were to forgo the IV, blood draw, cardiac monitor, or 12 lead as I had, he would be fired! If he pleaded the reasoning of his decision based on the seemingly clear history of the patient, hospital administration would say, "Well, Doctor, we don't really care what you think the patient's diagnosis is, you need to definitely rule out the possibility of an MI and all other potentially life-threatening differentials first, and then and only then do you get to make your diagnosis of esophageal reflux."

Defensive medicine is the logic behind the much more rigorous protocols in hospitals than for EMS. Somewhere along the way, more than one such presenting case, which seemed so obvious as to be a throwaway, ended up being dead wrong—literally. All for the allure of taking a short cut. Where is it written than a person with GERD cannot also have a heart attack? Not withstanding, a pretty large segment of the patient population, including experienced physicians, have complained of indigestion that ultimately ended up being an MI. So critical illnesses may not "always" be so easily identifiable. A little humility and caution can go a long way to avoiding disaster for these patients.

In addition to failing the patient medically, there's also the legal reality to consider. We're living in the age of the lawsuit. Billions of dollars in lost lawsuits have made hospitals risk averse. On the one hand, this has added to the cost of health care—in some instances, unnecessarily so—but it must be acknowledged that it has also significantly reduced morbidity and mortality (M&M).

In the interest of staying ahead of the curve, defensive medicine is a concept whose time has come for EMS. We have been living on borrowed time as far as lawsuits go. There have been some, but nowhere nearly as many as hospitals, doctors, and other medical providers. The reason is that in many areas of the country, EMS workers are still perceived to be volunteers or EMS personnel are simply ambulance drivers. But once we see the first high-priced case publicized, followed by the realization that most EMS agencies now carry million-dollar malpractice insurance, the floodgates could be opened.

Supervision, EMS style: EMS has never had any shortage of supervision by a whole hierarchy of line officers. These officers have always been there to ensure we wear our uniforms, wash our ambulances, and empty the trash regularly. But then when the alerting system activates, EMTs or paramedics jump into the ambulance, race down the street, and commence to practice medicine, many times under the most dire of circumstances, with no supervision whatsoever. It's really quite insane, if you stop to think about where the emphasis of supervision has been all this time. Are we in the building maintenance or vehicle-washing business or the emergency medicine business?

Given the lack of any meaningful medical supervision in many systems, it's inherently been left up to each and every individual provider to set his or her own standard of care. So an EMS agency of say thirty medics will end up operating under thirty different standards, which by definition is no standard at all. Since the inmates are running the asylum, those standards can (and, in fact, do) change based on whatever the individual medic happens to think is important or feels like doing at the moment. This phenomenon has typically been written off as the medic's "style." Paramedic Joe gives aspirin to every chest pain patient, whether it's a suspected cardiac or not. Paramedic Frank doesn't start IVs unless the patient is obviously critical. Paramedic Bob doesn't believe in CPAP. Amazing when you see it in print, isn't it? But this is exactly what's going on in many EMS systems to this day.

What other job in the world would a company hire people then let each and every individual employee decide for themselves what they felt like doing on any given day? Only EMS. K-Mart has more stringent job requirements for stock boys than many EMS systems have for their providers, and this is the life-and-death business of emergency medicine we're talking about. Ahhhh!

To err is human: In 1999, a white paper was published by the Institute of Medicine you may have heard of: *To Err Is Human—Building a Better Health Care System.* After extensive research, it estimated between 44,000 and 98,000 hospital patients die every year as a result of preventable medical errors. The report pointed out that even if the low number is correct, it still exceeds the death rates for motor vehicle accidents, breast cancer, and AIDS combined. Stunning, and keep in mind these fatal errors were in hospitals, staffed by the most educated and intelligent people in medicine, with systems comprised of large staffs of people, multiple levels of supervision, and specialized back-up available for IVs, intubations, respiratory therapy, and other interventions just a phone call away. So if that's the state of medicine in hospitals, you can't help but wonder what the treatment error rate is in EMS. But no one knows, because no one has ever looked.

All EMS systems are, of course, required to have a quality review process. But for all intents and purposes, in many states there are very few (if any) quality review requirements (beyond just having a process in place). Instead of trying to identify and correct problems before an incident, many quality improvement programs basically lay dormant until a complaint is filed, and then they swing into action.

Unlike the rest of medicine, which has nationalized oversight and enforcement by the Joint Commission on Accreditation of Healthcare Organizations (JACHO), there is no EMS equivalent. As a result, EMS is a patchwork of widely varying qualities, efficiencies, risks, and dangers, not only from state to state but region to region and even provider to provider.

In my home state of Pennsylvania, each EMS agency has an ambulance audit every three years, where a regional representative comes down and license ambulances based on whether they have state-required medical supplies and proper working equipment. Ironically, there is no state-mandated skills verification for EMS providers. The closest thing to an annual provider review in many systems is the medical director signing command forms, typically after just verifying the medic has acquired minimum continuing education (con-ed) credits and has a current CPR card. In many cases, ambulances and the equipment stocked in them are checked more thoroughly than the people who use them.

It doesn't take a prophet to realize that quality of patient care will eventually be mandated for EMS. We've already seen the beginning of quality targets being mandated by Medicare, whereby their reimbursements to hospitals will be based on their achieving certain quality care markers. For instance, if the "door to balloon (catheter) lab" time for an ST elevation myocardial infarction (STEMI) is greater than ninety minutes, Medicare will reimburse hospitals at a lower rate.

For all the complaints about insurance companies, it will ultimately be they and the pressure they bring to bear with financial incentives that will most dramatically improve the quality of health care. It will likely take several additional years, but at some point, this same market pressure will trickle down to EMS. The only question is whether your agency will get ahead of the curve now or be playing catch-up later.

CHAPTER 2

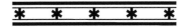

The Quality Improvement Coordinator

Lead, follow, or get out of the way.
—Thomas Paine

It doesn't take a genius: No one in EMS has a more critically important job than the quality improvement coordinator, and no one has a greater opportunity to make a difference on such a large scale.

It doesn't take a genius to be a great quality improvement coordinator, all it takes is dedication. Much of the work of quality improvement is tedious, unglamorous grunt work. But if you're willing to invest the time and effort, you can have a dramatic agency-wide impact on patient care.

Any provider who's been in EMS for any length of time knows the thrill of a successful resuscitation or turning the tide of impending death and delivering a patient to the hospital in better condition than they were found. That is an awesome achievement. It is also the very reason most of us got into EMS. But that's one call, one fleeting moment. You may ride that high for a while, but the next day it's ancient history.

Imagine being the first person to discover that an entire class of potentially critical patient, such as generalized weakness, frequently having their care downgraded. Imagine providing this valuable feedback to the providers and convincing them to increase their index of suspicion, resulting in a dramatic improvement in patient care across the board for your agency. Probably not as intense of a rush as being the greatest medic who ever lived (for a brief and shining moment) by saving a life, but all in all, a much greater impact on patient care than just one call. At that moment, you will know you made a difference. Identifying and correcting such problems will result in many more lives being saved on a continuous and ongoing basis. This is exactly what we did at Bucks County Rescue Squad and Central Bucks Ambulance in southeastern Pennsylvania.

Making a difference on a scale greater than one call at a time: Few people will ever have the opportunity of saving a human life. Fewer still will have the opportunity to improve the patient care of an entire system, resulting in the saving of countless lives. Your willingness to put the grunt work in, to effect such a massive and ongoing change as this, is the difference between management and leadership. Management has all too often become the art of maintaining the status quo and keeping things going as they are. And in the defense of management, when dealing with the day-to-day operation of an EMS agency, it does have a strong tendency to draw you in, pull you down, and demand a lot of your time just to put out all the brush fires. At the end of the day, most EMS officers are content with just keeping the operation going. Conversely, the quality improvement coordinator has an opportunity to focus directly on improving the operation and moving it forward to what EMS could and should be for the future.

There are many different EMS systems and agencies out there, all with their own history, dogma, and bureaucracies. Some quality coordinators want the job to get off the street, others take it as a promotion, and still others see it as a punishment. I know of an EMS provider from a nearby system to mine who was identified as being an outright danger to patients. On one particular call, this provider gave nitroglycerine to a patient complaining of chest pain . . . after the patient crashed his car into a bridge abutment and destroyed the steering wheel with his chest. The agency's response was to put this dangerous provider in charge of quality improvement. When someone asked why, in disbelief, the chief replied, "Can you think of a better way for her to learn?"

So, instead of putting one of the better providers in charge of quality improvement and directing them to try and pull the rest of the agency up to their level of proficiency, they opted to appoint a substandard provider and ran the risk of the derelict provider pulling the standard of care of the entire system down instead. The only saving grace is most quality coordinators are not activists, so their impact (for better or worse) is usually minimal.

Another popular way of choosing the quality coordinator is to tap the provider who's been on the job the longest, as if just showing up for twenty years imparts some kind of magical wisdom or proficiency.

Despite the best of intentions, many quality coordinators are prisoners of their systems. They take over their quality improvement program, and if they're lucky, they may receive a brief orientation by their predecessor, only to continue the failed or mediocre process that came before them. Rarely is any formalized training offered regarding how to administer a quality improvement program.

But whether you got to where you are by promotion, demotion, light duty, or blackmail, if you have the desire and you're not afraid of putting some time and effort into it, maybe even a little extra time and effort, you can make a difference.

The progressive quality improvement program we put in place at Bucks County Rescue Squad resulted in a 20 percent increase in the advanced life support (ALS) treatment rate within just three months; the program has been sustained for five years. Upon learning of this success, the other EMS agency I'm affiliated with, Central Bucks Ambulance, asked me if I would be willing to try and do the same for them. After I took over quality improvement at Central Bucks, I uncovered issues almost identical to those of Bucks County Rescue Squad, which only further reinforced the fact that in EMS, we all share most of the same problems. The first step to correcting any problem is to take a good hard, honest look at what's really going on below the surface and acknowledging those problems . . . or those opportunities for improvement.

But to see, you must first look.

CHAPTER 3

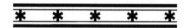

You Are Here

Improvise, adapt, overcome.
—Gunny Highway from the movie *Heartbreak Ridge*

You are here: Before implementing any new quality improvement program, you need to find out where you are. So the first thing I did at both agencies was take a few days to review all the patient care reports (PCRs) for the previous two months. The annual call volumes at Bucks County Rescue Squad and Central Bucks Ambulance were 3,600 and 4,200, or about 300 and 350 monthly calls, respectively. Although a lot of work, the volume was not prohibitive for a 100 percent PCR review.

Reviewing PCRs is a labor-intensive process, but it can reveal a wealth of information. With paper and pen in hand, I comprised a hit list of some of the more egregious deficiencies in care.

The undertreated and untreated: Some examples of downgraded care initially found included the following:

- Forty-eight-year-old male complaining of nausea, dyspnea on exertion and diaphoresis.
- Twenty-six-year-old, third trimester gravid female complaining of abdominal pain and tachycardic.
- Seventy-seven-year-old male complaining of generalized weakness and repeated falls.
- Eighty-year-old male, past medical history of cardiac and CVA, complaining of generalized weakness.

The last two examples of generalized weakness was repeated so many times I stopped counting. In many systems, generalized weakness is still dispatched as a basic life support (BLS) call, which only underscores how badly flawed and behind the times many of our systems still are. In my experience, generalized weakness is the most frequently undertreated and untreated chief complaint in EMS, despite the significant past medical histories of many of these patients and obvious potential for serious illness.

Patient refusals: Patient refusals are overall the greatest risk for lack of appropriate patient care, as well as the greatest potential for lawsuits. It's bad enough when a patient doesn't receive the most appropriate care by EMS prior to arrival at the hospital. It's even worse if they're left behind and receive no care at all. And that's exactly the picture opposing counsel will present in court. Consequently, patient refusals should be the single greatest concern of any quality coordinator.

Tally up the number of patient refusals, then divide that number by the total number of calls for the month; e.g., 45 refusals/250 calls = 18 percent. Although all refusals should be reviewed, the higher your refusal rate, the closer you may want to look. A 10 percent refusal rate is frequently cited as a national average, but there's no magic in any particular number. Only a detailed review of all calls within a given period will verify whether your patient refusal rate is appropriate or not.

You will likely find a lot of the aforementioned generalized weakness under either the patient refusal category or as patient assists or falls. These are the calls where the patient falls down and calls 911 for help up. Sometimes that's legitimately all that's needed. The problem is these patients are frequently not taken as seriously as they should. Many EMS providers will even openly complain of such calls being abuse of the EMS system.

A typical scenario is the crew arrives to find the patient on her back like a turtle. They pick the patient up, deposit her where she wants, sign here please, and leave. But an appropriate assessment is frequently never done. As previously mentioned, many and possibly even most of these calls may legitimately require nothing more than a lift assist. But keep in mind these are typically elderly patients with decreased mental acuity and sensibility to start with. They may not be aware of anything beyond, "I've fallen and can't get up." But they're not the medical professionals. We are.

EMS-initiated refusals: While most EMS providers are conscientious, some may require some guidance, and still others will require threat of termination to get them to do their job. LMS (Lazy Medic Syndrome) is an inevitable problem you will face. These are providers who will do anything to get out of doing their job, despite the risk to the patient and liability to the agency and themselves. Many of these lazy providers, left to their own devices for so long, have convinced themselves that EMS is "mostly" abused by the public, that most calls are not legitimate 911 calls, and that we're doing way too much of the hospital's job.

As with many problems, there are multiple contributing factors to quality of care issues in EMS. Burnout and fatigue resulting from many EMS providers working two and three jobs to make ends meet are two of them. Given the life-and-death business we're in, these are not acceptable excuses, but they are factors you need to be aware of.

Although it's beyond our control to modify the job market or give across-the-board raises so providers no longer have to work so many hours, there are some things we can do. Most notably, when the ambulances are checked out, housekeeping chores done, and any other shift required work completed, consider allowing providers to get some sleep if possible. As a result of medical error deaths due to fatigued interns, a few years ago New York became the first state to limit the number of hours interns can be on call. Many EMS systems are now confronted with similar problems with overworked, fatigued providers. It is certainly worth at least considering whether we shouldn't attempt to address this problem before a catastrophic incident propels some unfortunate agency into the feature story on *60 Minutes*.

One of the greatest risks with lazy or burnt-out medics is their handling of patient refusals. They will many times not only permit patients to refuse treatment, they will in many ways (subtle and not so subtle) encourage them to refuse. They do this by downplaying and explaining away potential problems or suggesting the patient could just drive himself to the hospital if he'd be more comfortable with doing that, thereby saving himself the expense of the ambulance bill.

After word got out about our quality improvement success, the quality coordinators from a few neighboring EMS agencies asked for help with their programs. At one agency, we discovered a 21 percent refusal rate, which means that one out of every five people who called 911 refused transport once the ambulance arrived. Many of these calls were suspicious based on how they were written. So if they were suspicious to me, you can just imagine how much fun a trial lawyer could have had with them. I confidentially interviewed the partners of some of the prime suspects and easily confirmed my suspicions. I resisted the impulse to kick the offenders up to the chief for disciplinary action. I did this for several reasons. First and foremost, because any true quality improvement program must be educational, not punitive (at least initially). Second, many providers have operated in a supervisory-free environment for so long they deserve the opportunity to change. And last, if you're fortunate enough to have providers willing to give you honest feedback from the trenches, you need to protect the confidentiality of these sources as much as possible.

You should also keep in mind the ultimate goal of any quality improvement program is the overall improvement of the entire system or agency, not getting unnecessarily distracted on a witch hunt. The exception to this rule is a recalcitrant provider who presents a significant or ongoing risk to patients. Determining when to move from education to discipline will be a judgment call for you to make.

If by now you've looked and haven't found problems similar to what I've described, congratulations are in order. You must be doing something right. Keep doing whatever it is you're doing, but read on anyway. It's likely there'll be an idea or two somewhere in this book that may help improve your patient care even further. If that isn't the case, then you need to sit down and write a book of your own on quality improvement.

Assuming you found deficiencies as I did, take your list of atrocities and schedule a meeting with your chief and medical director. Run down the list with them to educate them as to what's really going on out there, and watch their heads explode. Not unlike the phases of dealing with death, they'll likely run the gamut of denial, anger, resentment, and finally acceptance.

Reassure them that these results are unfortunately not uncommon in EMS and feel free to cite this book as a reference to that fact. Then tell them the good news; now that you've uncovered problems that no one could have imagined existed, you're going to fix the problems for them. All you need is their support in doing so. Please note, to make the most of this golden opportunity, you need the chief and medical director's undivided attention and willingness to support anything you want (within reason). So make sure you go to this meeting with a wish list in hand. If you need assistance, request the personnel; if you need dedicated time off the street, request it. If you need more money, forget it. There is no money in EMS.

CHAPTER 4

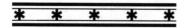

Quality Patient Care

Quality is not an act, it is a habit.
—Aristotle

Defining quality patient care. Every book written on the subject of quality invariably includes either a generic textbook definition or a tortured, all-encompassing made-up definition of quality. So here's mine: Quality patient care is simply providing the best patient care within your capability. That means giving every patient, from the cardiac arrest to the patient assist fall victim, the full benefit of your training, experience, and skill within the scope of your practice and resources available.

There's obviously no magic attached to my definition of quality patient care. It's perfectly acceptable and might not be a bad idea to come up with your own definition of quality patient care. Achieving success is much easier if you define what success is or at least set some benchmarks or goals you'd like to achieve.

Early ALS intervention: the best insurance policy. Early advanced life support monitoring and IV access is the best insurance policy against unanticipated events for at-risk patients. At-risk patients are those patients who are not obviously critical upon your arrival but have the potential to degenerate based on significant past medical history, an abnormal vital sign, or most commonly, a clue in the history of present illness. These are the patients who occasionally crash on you after you downgrade their care from ALS to BLS or two minutes after you drop them off at the ER. Or worse case scenario, you allow the patient to refuse treatment/transport without making a good faith effort to explain the risks and ramifications of doing so, and consequently, you end up right back there an hour or so later, typically for something that now is an obvious medical emergency.

When you take a step back and try to identify who these at-risk patients are, they're clearly the majority of patients who end up calling 911; chest pains, shortness of breath, syncope, and altered mental status are all pretty obvious. But as a mental exercise, let's look at it from the opposite side, as far as which patients you could reasonably and safely determine to *not* be at risk. Examples of clearly BLS patients would be minor lacerations with no major vessel involvement; other minor or isolated injuries such as simple extremity fractures or dislocations; short-term nausea, vomiting, and diarrhea; short-duration fever; and other such clearly noncritical cases. But even with simple fractures, there's the caveat if they're in significant pain, pain management could and should be offered if available.

There are many providers in EMS who do not deem pain management to be a part of their job. But I can assure you that any EMS provider who has fractured an ankle or had renal stones would likely be screaming for morphine or fentanyl. So why should our patients be made to suffer needlessly for another hour or even half hour, if we have the means to provide them with some relief? We need to constantly remind our providers that the "S" in EMS stands for service, service to our patient.

Moanings, groanings, and whinings: As you begin your noble quest to reduce morbidity and mortality to a greater degree than all others who have come before you, it's time for a reality check. Do not expect to be greeted as the visionary you are, hoisted up on the shoulders of your colleagues, or chauffeured around town for a ticker tape parade. Rather expect a more modest and subdued greeting, say more along the lines of the torches and pitchforks that greeted the monster of Dr. Frankenstein.

As you start to disturb the status quo and violate the EMS mantra of "Earn Money Sleeping," many providers may not like you so much. While you may improve the quality of care and reduce the pain and suffering of their patients, on the flip side you'll also be cutting into some providers' television watching and video game playing, asking them to do more work and possibly take computer-based training. You may even—God forbid—end up asking them to . . . read job-related material while on the clock. Oh, the humanity! But it is these negative connotations that will most immediately get the providers' attention. In the beginning, you will not be their favorite person. But over time, as you pull EMS into the modern age, saving more lives, ever so grudgingly, you probably will earn their respect.

Along the way, you can expect numerous sidebars with individual providers. Depending on your attitude, this experience could be anywhere from torture to dread to an opportunity to sell your programs on a more personal basis.

I can hear the arguments now. Actually I've heard them already, at both agencies where we initiated these programs. They were the same identical arguments at both places, which again reinforces the argument that, for the most part, EMS is pretty much the same all over. Why should we do the hospital's job for them? We're paramedics, we shouldn't be playing doctor. Too much advanced life support is bad. Treating the patient on the scene delays transport to the hospital. We could get sued for doing IVs that aren't clearly necessary. These were all actual arguments that were made by ALS providers.

Pathology is a dynamic process: Every veteran EMS provider, myself included, has boasted of our superhuman powers of being able to tell if a patient is sick just by a glance across the room. And many times you can. Unfortunately, the reverse it not true. You cannot tell someone is *not* sick just by looking at them.

Any medic that has been in EMS for any length of time has been dispatched for an ALS emergency, only to arrive to find a patient who seems perfectly fine with normal vital signs and good general appearance. And so, you opt to transport them BLS, only to have the patient either crash on the way to the hospital or right after you drop them off. And hopefully you at least wondered whether you missed something. Well, as far as vital signs or anything tangible at the exact moment of your physical exam, maybe not. The only clue may have been nothing more than the original reason the patient called 911: they fainted briefly, suddenly felt weak and fatigued, or experienced an unexplained episode of nausea and broke out in a sweat. By the time you arrived on the scene, many times that episode has resolved, with the patient fully recovered from the original insult. They could be back to feeling perfectly fine with normalized vital signs. They may even wonder whether they didn't over-react and question whether they should have called 911.

But pathology is a dynamic process. Onset can be acute or chronic; it can be a continuous progression, or symptoms may be intermittent as the body fights to maintain homeostasis. Sometimes that initial episode may be all the patient ever experiences; other times it will be the only warning there is of impending cardiovascular collapse. Therefore anyone who is concerned enough about a problem to call 911 needs to be taken seriously.

Index of suspicion: Being an EMS provider requires a certain degree of detective work. You can never assume anything just on face value. How many times have you yourself been dispatched for one reason and found the actual nature of the call to be something completely different? More than once, I myself have been dispatched for a fall victim only to arrive on the scene to find a cardiac arrest. Complete opposite ends of the medical spectrum, but both technically correct.

You don't win points in EMS by saving the patient the inconvenience of going to the hospital. You win points by identifying the not-so-obvious, elusive, or hidden medical problem or injury. A key point taught in the Basic Trauma Life Support course is that between 5 and 15 percent of seriously injured trauma patients will initially present with normal vital signs and no serious complaints. The secret to being a superstar in emergency medicine is not guessing right the most times, because no matter how many times you guess right, you'll be wrong every once in a while, and any one of those times could have grave consequences for your patient. That one wrong guess could also wipe out a thousand correct guesses on the tote board of EMS quality care.

The best way to approach every EMS call is to maintain a high index of suspicion, expect the unexpected, always err on the side of caution, and always be willing to look a little deeper just to be sure. You can have the lowest IQ legally allowable by law to be an EMS provider and still be a paramedical genius if you do nothing more than maintain a high index of suspicion and err on the side of caution with your patients.

The gold standard of EMS is to over-triage medical patients to ALS for the same reason we over-triage trauma patients to trauma centers: so we don't miss anything. Obvious life threats are . . . well, obvious; many other serious illnesses are not always so obvious. The goal of progressive EMS, just as Johnny and Roy in the 1970s TV show *Emergency* once explained to a patient, is to bring the hospital to the patient. As opposed to making the patient wait and suffer further, untreated, during transport.

Only a fool waits for the patient to explode in front of them before acknowledging the potential for a critical illness or injury. Pushing a high index of suspicion is probably the single most important aspect in improving your agency's standard of care.

Generalized weakness: At both agencies where I coordinate the quality improvement program, I have found that generalized weakness is by far the most commonly undertreated type of call.

There are of course plenty of things generalized weakness could be—some of them are life threatening, many others are not. But can you really pick out the critical ones from the noncritical ones based on just a pulse rate, blood pressure, and glance across the room? The answer is, No! And neither can the best emergency medicine physician with a whole lot more education than you, which is why they'll order blood draws, X-rays, ECGs, and all sorts of other diagnostics. Yet there is no shortage of EMS providers who would not hesitate to go where any doctor would fear to tread. They routinely do this by downgrading the care of their patients based on a single set of vital signs, taken at a moment in time and totally discounting everything the patient is telling them.

If a patient is usually able to function appropriately but is suddenly now falling, this could be the only hint there is of a stroke, cardiac arrhythmia, infarct, infection, or electrolyte derangement. Continuing to pick the patient up, plopping him back into his chair or bed, and then leaving without a much more in-depth and thoughtful assessment is unethical, immoral, and dangerous. Not infrequently, providers will be called back for the same patient numerous times. This may be a red flag in and of itself that you missed something the first time around.

In addition to the standard vital signs of pulse, respiratory rate, and blood pressure, the following advanced diagnostics should be considered for any patient complaining of weakness:

- Cincinnati stroke screen
- Blood glucose check
- Cardiac monitor to rule out arrhythmia
- 12-lead ECG (if available) to rule out ischemia or infarct
- Blood draw (if accepted by the receiving hospital) to check cardiac enzymes, electrolytes, and other blood chemistry

EMS vs. a taxi ride: Some will argue there's a lot of things the hospital will do that EMS won't. They're the hospital; we're just the means to get the patients to the hospital. A fair enough argument for debate. But it all comes down to how you view yourself and your profession. Many in EMS today still cling to the antiquated mentality of "load and go" for all patients and all occasions—a quick ride to the hospital and dumping more untreated patients into the increasingly overburdened ER. Those who make the argument of "load and go" must assume the burden of explaining how it is then that EMS has not progressed and why we should not be doing more for our patients than thirty years ago, despite the addition of thousands of dollars' worth of advanced technology, purchased with the obvious expectation that it would be put to some use. The reality is that the "load and go" style of EMS for patients we are capable of treating is no better patient care than what the patient could get with a taxicab (and for a lot less money).

Most advanced life support units now carry the initial diagnostics and first line treatments for most medical emergencies. So why haul patients and all this high-priced equipment around and rush to the hospital, when we can do all the first things the hospital will do, despite the fact that we can do it sooner and quicker, since we only have one patient to their many? The only reason to be rushing patients to the hospital in this day and age is for those patients experiencing time-sensitive medical emergencies we are not capable of treating, such as trauma patients who could require surgical intervention or stroke patients who may qualify for revascularization.

Patient denial: No one wants to believe they could be seriously ill or dying. Patient denial is a well-established and well-documented phenomenon. It's human nature and to be expected. EMS providers are medical professionals and emergency medicine experts (or at least that's how the public perceives us). As the highest medical authority of the 99.999 percent of the earth's surface that is not a hospital or physician's office, the patient will look to the EMS provider for validation that there is nothing wrong. Tempting though it may be, EMS providers must not allow themselves to be drawn into the patient's denial. Our job is to play the devil's advocate and err on the side of caution, which is treat and transport anything that looks, feels, or smells like a potentially serious medical problem.

Patient assists and falls: One type of call that causes more moans and groans than any other is the patient assist. The typical scenario is an elderly patient who has "fallen and can't get up." You respond to the call, possibly non-emergently (and maybe taking the scenic route to boot). You arrive, possibly with your annoyance obvious. You pick the patient up and return her to her original upright position, get her to sign the release form, and off you go.

Geriatric patients are a real assessment challenge. In addition to reduced mental acuity and sensibility, which comes with age, these patients typically have a myriad of medical problems that can further erode their perception and sensation such as diabetes, Alzheimer's, or a previous stroke. Additionally, many of these patients will be on a host of medications, which while effective in treating specific medical problems, may also have side effects that further decrease their sensibility, such as analgesics. Antidepressants and other psychotropic medications may also decrease their strength, balance, and awareness.

Despite all this potential, the very simple but key question is frequently never asked: did you slip, trip, or lose your footing and fall, or did you get dizzy, weak, feel faint, or pass out and fall? But as a matter of practicality, your index of suspicion must extend beyond even those patients with the right answer to this question. While writing this book, I was dispatched to a BLS fall victim. I arrived to find a seventy-year-old female who appeared to be in otherwise good health, lying on the sidewalk in no apparent distress and moving all extremities. She denied being injured or striking her head, and there were no obvious signs of trauma. When I put the question above to her, she said she just slipped and fell and couldn't get back up. But it immediately seemed suspicious to me that someone capable of walking outside on her own could fall but then not be capable of getting back up after several minutes. We assisted her first to sit up and then stand. She said she was fine and just wanted to go home. But as soon as she tried to walk away, we immediately noticed an obvious ataxic (uncoordinated) gait. On further questioning, she did not know what year it was, her address, or birth date. Sometimes the patient might not legitimately know or be aware of what caused their fall. This makes perfect sense if you consider the possibility that the same underlying central nervous system insult causing the weakness or lack of coordination could very easily also cause altered mental status. In this case, the patient was transported to the hospital where she was diagnosed with a stroke of the cerebellar region of her brain—the area of the brain which controls coordination.

The key to evaluating weakness, falls, and patient assists is first and foremost not to start out assuming everything is okay, but rather the complete opposite: assuming there's an underlying medical cause for the fall and objectively evaluate further to either confirm or disprove it. If you can get through a reasonably thorough assessment and not be as suspicious as when you started and feel comfortable leaving the patient, then—and only then—should you allow them to sign off.

The two-minute EMS challenge: Beyond deploying the EMS safety net to ensure all critical and potentially critical patients receive the benefit of advanced care, it should not be too much to expect in twenty-first-century EMS that providers perform a rapid but purposeful patient assessment to identify these patients. This may sound simple enough, and you may even be under the impression that it's being done, but jump on an ambulance or show up on a few calls and see if it really is happening and happening consistently. You may be surprised.

Upon showing up on a near syncope call not too long ago, I observed, two providers alternate questions as one provider reached for a radial pulse. As they continued taking the patient's history, the other provider retook the same pulse a couple minutes later. Not uncovering any reason not to, the providers eventually allowed the patient to walk to the ambulance. About nine minutes later, the providers finally got around to taking a full set of vital signs. The temptation of taking short cuts such as this in patient assessments is not uncommon. The mistaken belief is that by not doing a complete patient assessment up front, it will somehow save time. But if you stand back and witness this philosophy at work, you realize it not only doesn't save time, it actually wastes time by incomplete, redundant, and delayed actions. Delays in identifying a serious underlying problem will result in the delay of treating the problem.

Some providers and crews are more efficient than others; some providers do preplan or decide who will do what ahead of time, but that may be the exception rather than the rule. And few EMS systems have an official policy for something that seems so obvious as to not be necessary. Conversely, all hospitals have a clear policy whereby any patient who reaches triage or a bed automatically has a full set of vitals signs taken, including temperature, whether they look or feel febrile or not. Vital signs may be taken by the nurse or, increasingly, by ER technicians. A nurse or physician will then take the patient history and perform a focused examination.

As previously mentioned, a patient can have a potentially life-threatening illness or condition such as a dysrhythmia and look perfectly fine and be stone cold stable while sitting there talking to you. Based solely on that general impression, it might seem reasonable to have the patient walk to the ambulance rather than carry them. But jumping to that conclusion without performing an appropriate assessment could result in an unconscious (or worse) patient you may then have to carry by hand. While this scenario involves a small number of patients, it clearly can and does happen, but it should not happen.

Mandating by official policy that all medical patients receive a rapid patient assessment similar to what is now standard of care for trauma patients has the potential for significant improvement in quality of patient care. You can't treat what you don't know exists. The policy should assign clear roles. An example might be provider number one (e.g., the driver or EMT on an ALS unit) will immediately take a full set of vital signs, attached the cardiac monitor, and perform a 12-lead ECG if warranted. Provider number two (e.g., the primary care provider) will at the same time take a history and perform a focused exam based on the chief complaint. If a two-person crew works together in such a coordinated fashion, they should know everything they initially need to know about the patient, mainly whether the patient was critical or potentially critical, requires immediate intervention, or as in most cases, can wait for any interventions to be initiated until they're either in the ambulance or en route to the hospital. This coordinated team approach to rapid patient assessment is what I've come to call the Two-Minute EMS Challenge.

Clearly defined roles leave nothing to the imagination as far as expectations. Identifying critical and potentially critical patients is most times the weak link in the chain. But if you think about it, it's also literally job number one in EMS. Once providers know the actual condition of the patient, for the most part they will make reasonable decisions on whether critical interventions need to be initiated immediately, wherever they happen to be, or can wait until they're in the ambulance or on the way to the hospital if the patient is stable. But all good medicine begins with a comprehensive patient assessment.

Attitude is everything: One aspect of extraordinary patient care that is frequently overlooked is attitude. No matter what it is you do, your attitude and demeanor will always show through.

EMS is not law enforcement, and our patients are not the enemy, despite the fact that some providers treat them that way. Although just another routine call for us, it's frequently a major life event for our patients and their families. Many things said in the course of a call will be replayed in the minds of our patients and their families over and over again and will forever be what EMS is to them.

I had a call a couple years ago where I learned one of the most valuable lessons of my career. It was change of shift, and my oncoming partner and I were dispatched for an abdominal pain call before we ever got a chance to check out our ambulance. Everything seemed to be either missing or disorganized. Once things start poorly on a call, it's frequently difficult to turn it around. I blew the IV and just couldn't seem to get anything done right. It was a horrible call. Fortunately, it was not a critical call. But to my amazement, when we got to the hospital, the patient was grateful and more appreciative than most successful resuscitations I've had. The patient thanked me for what she called the best care she'd ever gotten by EMS. I was dumbfounded. On the ride back to squad headquarters, I had an epiphany. I had been nice to the patient, and that was apparently what mattered most to her. Then I realized, I have always gotten far more compliments, thank yous, and expressions of heartfelt appreciation over the years for how I treated my patients, rather than the treatments I gave to them (what in the rest of medicine is known as bedside manner).

Fairly or not, you will be judged more by your demeanor than anything else. Patients and their families will also be more appreciative to you for showing concern, kindness, and compassion than for successfully completing the most impressive and difficult lifesaving intervention.

That's pretty confounding to most of us in EMS, because it's the complete opposite of what we believe the priorities of EMS to be. The good news is that your attitude and how you choose to treat people is 100 percent within your control (and a lot easier than intubating a grade-four airway). Shortly after we made providers aware of this little pearl of wisdom, we experienced a noticeable influx of thank you cards and letters, which by far exceeded anything the agency had ever seen before.

The fact is most people have little knowledge of what a normal blood pressure is or what tombstone elevation on an EKG means. But most people can instinctively tell whether the person caring for them cares about them, and that is very comforting and reassuring to them at a time when they probably need it the most.

Think about how you feel when you go to see your family doctor. Family practitioners typically present as confident, professional, and genuinely caring. The best will even seem to take a personal interest in you. The result of their demeanor makes you feel safe, secure, and reassured. Now keep in mind you were most likely seeing your doctor for a cold, a sore throat, or a stomach virus. So imagine how much more important your bedside (or curbside) manner is to a patient during a medical emergency, real or imagined.

If you're still not convinced of how important bedside manner can be, I'll challenge you to conduct a little experiment. Once you've completed your assessment and initial treatments on a noncritical patient and you're transporting him, strike up a casual conversation with him (while keeping an eye on the cardiac monitor). Many times you'll notice the patient's heart rate decrease as you distract him from his problem and put him at ease. This is especially true if you happen to engage him in conversation about a subject of interest or passion to him. Physiology 101: decreased heart rate equals less cardiac workload, equals less myocardial oxygen demand, equals overall patient improvement. Many times you can pick up the perfect topic for your patient by a glance around the home, noticing such things as sports or military memorabilia or books on a certain topic.

CHAPTER 5

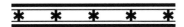

Prescription for Progress

Every question has an answer, every problem has a solution.
—Joe Hayes, Author

|

No-fault quality improvement: In the 1970s, the airline industry learned a valuable yet costly lesson regarding discipline in quality improvement. An airline pilot made an error, resulting in a near-miss. The airline responded to the mishap by suspending the pilot. A few months later, a pilot with another airline made the same error, this time resulting in a crash, with all onboard being killed. So is discipline an effective tool in quality management? No. It only encourages people to cover up their errors and does nothing to correct the underlying problem. If one person can make an error, others can and will, unless appropriate changes are made to the process, the equipment, or the behavior of the personnel.[1]

Any progressive quality improvement program must be no-fault (at least initially). In other words, providers should not be punished for honest, non-malicious errors. The reality is as long as human beings are a part of any system, there will always be errors in the system. One of the goals of the quality improvement coordinator should be to enlist the help of providers to identify problems and potential problems and correct them before they generate a complaint, result in harm, or get you sued.

Kick-off: In order to begin anything new, you gotta have a kick-off or a well-publicized beginning. If the troops don't know there's a new expectation or change in policy, you won't see much of a change in behavior. The more prominent and high profile the kick-off, the more impact you have coming out of the gate. The best way to do this is with as much fanfare and in as many different ways as possible. The more people are bombarded with the same message, the more impact the message will have.

If you have employee meetings or any kind of formalized shift change roll call, this would be a good time to put the word out. In addition to the live, all-hands-on-deck approach, the kick-off should be further echoed in as many other ways as possible, such as posting notices and memos in each provider's mailbox (electronic and physical). The more you consistently

---

[1]   1. O'Connor RE., Fairbanks RJ. et al. Reducing adverse events in EMS. *Improving Quality in EMS*. 2nd ed. Ed. Swor RA., Pirrallo RG. Kendall Hunt Publishing; 2005, 154

repeat the same message, the more likely it will be remembered. One final note: to get a message across to people, keep it short, sweet, and to the point. The reality is, when it comes to memos and posted announcements, most adults have an attention span only slightly longer than a two-year-old. The most effective memos and announcements are ideally no more than a few sentences, highlighted with large, BOLD print, which states the case.

Let them know you're watching: The very first thing I did after completing my baseline analysis was to publicize the start of the new quality improvement program. To emphasize the need for it, I posted the same list of patient care issues I showed the chief and medical director. I feel it's only fair to show the providers the same data that management sees. In fact, in the final analysis, it's probably more valuable to show the providers the problems you encounter than management, since they're the ones who ultimately have the capacity to correct the problems.

In addition to showing the need for change, I also advertised the fact that we would immediately begin doing a 100 percent patient care report review for all providers. While it may not be very flattering, the fact is most people will perform better if they know they're being watched. This is probably the fundamental reason why management positions exist in every business.

Educational, not punitive: Most importantly to the sense of self-preservation of the providers, don't forget to emphasize that the new quality improvement program is "no-fault." The only goal is identifying and correcting problems. Ultimately it's educational, not punitive. If a provider is deviating from protocol, not doing something they're supposed to be doing or doing something they shouldn't be doing with regard to patient care, the first step in most cases should be to try and educate them as to how and why they should be doing things.

If providers believe they're being watched and will not be penalized for an honest mistake, you've effectively removed the two biggest obstacles to problem identification and resolution. Despite the theory of all this, no one was more surprised than I was when I actually starting getting phone calls from providers. One provider called me in the middle of the night to inform me that in the heat of the moment, they failed to put a c-collar on a patient with a suspected mechanism of injury. Another provider called to inform me that they realized after the fact that they were too slow in getting the pacer pads on a prearrest bradycardia.

Provider awareness: The most important effect of a provider having to respond to a letter of inquiry or calling to report a problem is probably the discomfort of having to do so. Although I'm not a psychologist, there can be little doubt that that discomfort probably does more to prevent errors from being repeated than anything else.

Redefining our role: In the beginning, paramedics were told to go forth, treat immediate and obvious life threats, and transport all others without getting fancy. That was thirty years ago. In many systems, including the author's, no formal change in marching orders has ever been clearly disseminated, despite the fact that we have since had our protocols amended to include such non-emergent treatments as pain management, as well as nausea and vomiting. But in many cases, no one has officially explained the expanding role of EMS to the providers. Consequently, there are many old medic holdouts and some new medics who choose to practice minimal EMS, who believe their job is still to do nothing more than treat only immediate and obvious life-threatening emergencies.

Lack of leadership here may largely be due to the fragmented world of many EMS systems. The protocols are there, but in many cases the state delegates to the regions and the regions delegate to the individual agencies to set and enforce the actual standard of care. Many agencies decline assuming active leadership on standard of care, believing it's the state's or region's role. The result is, "the buck stops over there," with all the different echelons of EMS waiting for all the other echelons to establish a standard of care. While some agencies have taken the initiative to set a progressive standard of care, many have by default left it up to each and every individual provider to decide for themselves what the standard of care should be, which as previously mentioned is not a standard.

Protocols without a clearly defined standard of care are merely suggestions. In many cases, I've found the minimalist providers opt to load and go and drop off more untreated patients into the already overburdened ER.

Setting the standard of care: Well, if you haven't run away screaming by now, tag, you're it! So to whatever degree the standard of care has not been clearly established by your state, region, or agency, it's now up to you.

The two main objectives of any successful quality improvement program are improving the quality of care and standardizing care. In other words, the quality of care a patient receives should not be dependent upon which EMS provider they happen to get. A patient with suspected ischemic chest pain should receive the same appropriate care regardless of which shift happens to respond.

The core business: Any EMS agency not 100 percent dedicated to striving to provide the highest quality of patient care should not be in the business of emergency medicine. Many agencies, in addition to providing EMS to their community, also provide additional services such as bike teams, strike teams, urban search and rescue teams, tactical EMS, and so on. But your primary obligation is your core business—the emergency medical service the public depends on you to provide. If your agency has been distracted from their primary responsibility by these peripheral functions, it's time to ensure you're performing your primary mission adequately. One caveat, with regard to any of the above-mentioned additional services, they should also be included in the quality review process. You should also ensure that they are maintaining some kind of patient care documentation. Since these auxiliary functions are off the radar of the main business, they frequently fall through the cracks, and you could end up with providers medicating or shocking patients with no documentation. If any of those cases happen to be legally challenged for any reason and you have no documentation, you might as well just ask opposing counsel very nicely how much they'll take to go away and write them a check. But that won't be the end of it. The next thing you can expect is a visit from the folks from the state and region to investigate your operation. But even that won't be all. The most likely painful thing of all will be the very unkind headlines that will appear in your local newspaper, with no mention of all the good you've done and the countless lives you've saved over the years. An ounce of prevention is worth a ton of damage control.

A noble profession: There is no more noble profession in the world than saving lives, and that's what we do. People go to the movies and watch TV dramas with actors pretending to do what we do for real. In the day-to-day grind of doing our job, we sometimes forget just how extraordinary we really are. There's something unique about a person who can handle any kind of emergency, save a life, and occasionally even raise the dead and call it just another day at the office.

No one came into EMS for the money, and God knows, it's unlikely we'll ever get paid what we deserve in this lifetime, but pride in a difficult job well done can be very personally rewarding and a good management tool. A good quality improvement coordinator should never miss an opportunity to stroke the pride of the providers for the extraordinary job they do. This segues perfectly into emphasizing the moral obligation to always do their best, no less than any doctor would.

Selling quality one conversation at a time: Casual conversations are an excellent way of selling a new and improved quality improvement program on a more personal level, one provider at a time. You can't ask a protocol or policy question, and the reasoning and logic behind some changes may not always be clear to everyone, especially when they run counter to years of precedent. Providers can ask you questions, and you can make the case and maybe remind them of the real purpose of EMS. Many providers have gotten so caught up in either the paycheck or the thrill of the occasional critical call that they've forgotten that the main reason we're here is for the patient, no matter what type of call.

To prepare you for the onslaught of providers awakened from their lethargic slumber, I've included a few of the most frequently asked questions, and my best responses.

Q: Won't doing more advanced life support extend our on-scene time?

A: Based on the results at the two similar-sized agencies where I'm the quality coordinator, the additional interventions of an IV, blood draw, and cardiac monitor added between just five and seven minutes to the typical 911 call. If you're doing all of these first line interventions (that will eventually need to be done anyway), it's not wasting time. It's also not delaying care, it's advancing care. And as previously mentioned, if you're able to get those interventions done fifteen to thirty minutes sooner, as opposed to waiting for the hospital to do them, it's the best, easiest, and cheapest insurance policy you'll ever have against anything unforeseen going wrong. If the patient crashes, you're ready. Well worth the few extra minutes.

Q: We're just five or ten minutes out from the hospital. Why does it matter whether we get an IV in a few minutes sooner?

A: Well, it's not just five or ten minutes, as frequently cited. That's just the transport time. The patient contact time is typically two to three times that, in addition to the transport time. Plus, it's not like the minute you wheel the patient into the ER, IV lines drop out of the ceiling and start on these patients. We have one patient; the ER's in most cases have dozens. Unless the patient is clearly critical, it could easily be fifteen minutes to half an hour before the patients gets the first line interventions we could have started much sooner.

Q: Why should we do the nurse's job when they get paid more than us?

A: We're not doing the nurse's job, we're doing our job. We're just trying to do it better than we did before. True, if we start providing IV life lines and monitoring to every patient who could benefit from it instead of just those who are in obvious dire need of it, we'll end up doing some IVs and blood draws the ER nurses otherwise would have done. But beyond having to do five to seven more minutes of actual work ourselves or worrying about who might be getting away with something, the focus of any true medical professional should be doing what is in the best interest of the patient.

Q: We're paramedics; we should only be treating immediate life threats and transporting the rest to the hospital for definitive care.

A: Well, if we were still back in the 1970s you'd be correct. But since then we've added thousands of dollars of advanced medical equipment, as well as non-emergent protocols for pain management and nausea and vomiting. So the expectation must be that we should be providing more patient care instead of just giving patients a taxi ride to hospital.

Q: We're not doctors, there's no need to treat everybody who calls 911.

A: No, we're not doctors. They work in a big building that doesn't rock and roll while they're trying to treat their patients. They have a staff of nurses and technicians to help treat their patients. They also have specialist back-ups in every category; respiratory therapy, IV team, anesthesiology, and so on to come to their rescue when things go south.

We have our partners. In the streets, it's us against the world. No back-up, no safety net, no excuses. You either get the job done or you don't. If you don't get the job done on a critical call, the patient dies.

So, if you want an easy job, go work in a hospital, otherwise take pride in being one of a special breed of people who can be thrown into any situation and get the job done no matter what. And take pride in being the best at what you do.

CHAPTER 6

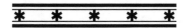

Retrospective Quality Improvement

If you want something you've never had before, you have to be willing to do something you've never done before.
—Drina Reed

Retrospective: adj., from the Latin, where "retro" means "after" and "spective" means "to look or see." Reviewing PCRs is tedious and arduous work. But physicians and many other people in medicine have been known to read massive amounts of material without their eyes falling out and their heads exploding. As the epigraph above intones, if you want to achieve results nobody ever has before, you have to be willing to do more than anyone else ever has before.

Fairly or not, the quality of care a patient receives will most often be judged by the PCR. Because long after the call is done and forgotten, the PCR is all that lives on.

The more PCRs you review, the better insight you will gain into the quality of care your agency is providing, as well as the job your individual providers are doing. But as you look behind the curtain, be prepared to view reality for the first time. Some providers who are believed to be God's gift to EMS may quickly be exposed as being quite humanly flawed. Some providers who are thought to be nervous and gun-shy may prove to be thorough and diligent providers. Besides some surprises, you'll also see all of the blemishes. It will not always be pretty, but remember these problems were always there, they're just now being seen for the first time. The importance of this first step cannot be overstated, because the first step in resolving any problem is recognizing and acknowledging that the problem exists.

100 percent quality review: As soon as I took over as quality improvement coordinator, I jumped right in with both feet. Knowing nothing about quality improvement, I secluded myself in an upstairs office with months' worth of paper PCRs piled high on the desk. Several hours later, the chief came to see what happened to me. "What are you doing?" he asked, incredulously. "Reviewing the charts," I replied. "All of them?" he asked. "Yeah, isn't that what I'm supposed to be doing?" "No!" he exclaimed. He opened the center drawer and handed me the region's call review criteria. "You just need to look at a portion of them," he explained, "mandatory review type calls such as cardiac arrests, Medevac flights, and level one traumas and just a percentage of all other random calls."

At that point, I only had a couple weeks of PCRs left, so I decided to finish. When I was done, I looked at the list of issues I identified by reviewing all PCRs and compared them with the region's call review criteria. Ninety percent of all the issues I uncovered—many major—would never have been discovered had I followed the region's criteria. Taking one step back, it was easy to see why. All the emphasis was clearly placed on the high-intensity, high-profile calls. All the remaining calls, the "routine" calls, which were also the majority of calls, were frequently trivialized. But upon review, they were anything but trivial (or being appropriately handled). Abdominal pain and generalized weakness are not sexy or exciting, but they have quite a bit of potential to be critical: MI, aneurysm, and acute gastritis are a few possibilities for abdominal pain, and hypoglycemia, sepsis, and MI are some causes for generalized weakness. The seriousness of many of these patients was frequently not appreciated, sometimes despite several red flags indicating the patient was already in extremis.

This was my first realization that conventional standards in quality improvement might leave a lot to be desired. Consequently, based on the results of my review, I decided as long as I had the time, I would do a 100 percent retrospective review. I've made the time ever since, reviewing an average of 300 calls a month at Bucks County Rescue Squad and about 350 calls a month at Central Bucks Ambulance. That's a lot of PCRs to read, but it's resulted in a great return on investment. Like anything else in life, the more you put into an effort, the more you will get out of it.

If you cannot review 100 percent of your total calls, you absolutely need to at least do 100 percent provider review; that is, review as many PCRs as you can of each of your providers, and do not just limit it to the high-intensity, high-profile calls. I'm confident you will find, as I have, that the greatest value of a retrospective review will be found by reviewing the more common calls, such as abdominal pain, generalized weakness, and patient assists. Medics are much more easily motivated to do an excellent job on the more glamorous, dire emergencies. But the true mark of a professional provider is how they handle the routine call.

Advertise 100 percent review: Regardless of whether you do 100 percent call volume review or 100 percent provider review, advertise the fact that you are doing 100 percent quality review. Knowing they're being watched is a great motivator to do a good job, for self-preservation if no higher moral purpose.

True leaders: If your call volume is so large that 100 percent provider review cannot physically be done by one person, consider asking for additional personnel to assist. It's always good to have at least one back-up for any job anyway. If you should leave, quit, or die, all the effort and progress you've made should not die with you. Being truly committed to improving patient care is the noblest of causes. You may never get the recognition you deserve for what you achieve, but you'll know and so will all those close to you. All true leaders put the mission first.

Convenience counts: Where is it written that a job must be inconvenient to count or one must suffer for one's work like an artist? Because of the greater benefit attached to reviewing as many PCRs as possible, if there's any way you can make it easier or more convenient for yourself, do it.

In the beginning, I reviewed paper charts—stacks and stacks of them. In the process, after several months of reviewing a hundred pounds of charts printed off from a computer-based system, I suggested, and it was quickly agreed to, to stop printing off PCRs unless there was a specific request or reason. This has saved countless trees and some money too. If you can access your PCR data system at your convenience by a laptop—either your agency's or your own (with authorization)—it will greatly increase the number of PCRs you'll be able to review.

Peer review: The retrospective review process begins with a peer review, in which I audit PCRs. I look for the following main items on each PCR:

- Patient age
- Past medical history
- Patient medications
- Chief complaint
- Exam and physical finding
- Treatments

I never look at the provider's names until after the review of the PCR is complete to avoid any prejudice on my part.

I cast a wide net in my peer review, pulling any PCR that looked exceptionally well managed, poorly managed, difficult to manage, as well as any unusual or complicated calls and calls of interest. I also noted any cases where there were multiple responses to the same address or same patient for closer scrutiny.

Keep in mind, even though the retrospective review is typically administrative and not time sensitive, if you discover a critical issue such as an ongoing practice that could be dangerous to either the patient or providers, do not hesitate to alert operations or providers immediately.

An excellent example of this was when we noticed a series of unsecured combative patients being transported. There is nothing more dangerous to the patient or the EMS crew than transporting an out-of-control patient in the back of a moving ambulance, with only half your personnel there to control the patient while the other half is driving. We quickly identified the problem as failure on the part of many providers to consider sedation for combative patients. The problem was quickly resolved by simply reminding the providers that patient sedation is a safer alternative—for both the patient and the provider—than a wrestling match in the back of a moving ambulance.

Additionally, if you notice repeat responses to the same address for similar complaints that could be indicative of an environmental emergency, such as carbon monoxide poisoning, once again do not hesitate to take immediate action. You may be the only person who gets to see the big picture, especially if the repeat calls span multiple shifts. This underscores the added benefit of early review of PCRs, ideally being done on a daily basis, resources and time permitting.

Call feedback: If you're doing something wrong or if there's a better way to do something and no one ever tells you, how would you ever know?

EMS in Bucks County was all volunteer back when I started in 1980. We were all out to be the best, and we all thought we were. But now that I look back with the benefit of 20/20 hindsight, I'm much more skeptical. We completed our abbreviated training, hit the streets, and continued to do what little we were taught to do. All the motivation and desire in the world cannot compensate for lack of knowledge. And how much knowledge of anatomy, physiology, and pathophysiology of everything that could possibly go wrong with the human body and the progression of signs and symptoms can possibly be squeezed into just nine months (or even twenty-four months of training, for that matter)? If it were all that encompassing, physicians would be starting off or ending their medical training in a medic class.

Because much of our profession does not presently allow for more training or longer preceptorships, a progressive, continuous quality improvement program is probably the next best thing to try to bridge the gap.

Medical director involvement: Without a doubt, most of the success of the quality improvement programs at both Bucks County Rescue Squad and Central Bucks Ambulance was due to strong medical direction involvement. Once a month, I meet with the medical director at each agency to review any issues I uncovered during my retrospective peer review.

I present any good, bad, questionable, and interesting cases I discovered to the medical directors as they review the PCR for details. The quality coordinator has the knowledge of scope of practice, current protocols, and peer perspective. The medical director has a much broader and more in-depth knowledge of medicine in general and emergency medicine in particular. For educational purposes, this is invaluable. Remember, quality improvement is about improving quality. If the only knowledge base you have to build your improvement on is from the same, relatively low level of medicine such as another medic, the amount of improving you'll be capable of doing will be extremely limited. Feedback from someone with more knowledge is the ideal way to learn from calls, particularly difficult or problem calls, and raise the bar of patient care.

External issues: Any PCR or incident report where there appears to be a problem external to the agency should also receive scrutiny. An all-encompassing quality improvement system does not stop with the agency's providers.

If there is a lack of cooperation with police or fire departments, interdepartmental communication (and possibly even a liaison) should be established. Establishing communication between agency heads or other designated officers, conducting multiagency drills, or even organizing meet-and-greets to get to know people you're going to be working with (before you're thrown together in the heat of battle) can go a long way to fostering cooperation. If a first responder, firefighter, police officer, or nursing home attendant has been identified as doing something contrary to the appropriate standard of patient care, we have an obligation as the highest authority of prehospital medical providers to try and correct the problem. The most obvious way to do this is alert the other agency of the issue and try to suggest a correction to the problem, *diplomatically* (not in front of the patient or witnesses).

As an example, say it has been noticed that nursing home staff continually place respiratory distress patients on four liters O_2 by face mask. You should consider alerting nursing home management of the potential danger of this practice. The correspondence could review the mechanics of the problem, such as such low flow O_2 coupled with the patient's airway being partially occluded by the mask results in a lot of the exhaled CO_2 being retained and rebreathed by the patient. You could point out how this practice could lead to hypoxia and potentially even death for the already compromised respiratory patient.

Emphasis must again be stressed that the wording of any external correspondence should be nonaccusatory, educational, and diplomatic. Also, before taking on the world, make sure to get the approval of management. Additionally, any such correspondence will carry much more clout if the medical director reviews and signs the correspondence. There of course is no guarantee, regardless of how diplomatic and right you are, that any external agency will respond positively to a suggestion made by you. But your moral obligation has been met, having tried.

Be sure to retain a copy of any external correspondence. You may want to let them know you're keeping a file by printing "copy to file" at the bottom. You also may want to consider forwarding a copy of the correspondence to a superior within the agency, such as chief operating officer or medical director, or an overseeing agency, such as the county or state department of health. Whoever else you copy correspondence to, be sure to note it on the bottom of the correspondence. Doing the right thing because they think they're being watched is not just limited to EMS providers.

CHAPTER 7

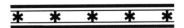

Concurrent Quality Improvement

It's all right to try and fail, but you should never fail to try.
—Richard Nixon

Concurrent: occurring at the same time. A progressive quality improvement program should be an active, engaged process, before, during, and after the call.

While retrospective quality review is an important part of the quality improvement process, it should not be the whole process. Theoretically, you could sit down and write a PCR for a totally fictitious call without ever leaving your seat, and as long as you didn't include anything too bizarre, no one would ever know. You'd have to be pretty naive to think that falsification of documentation, to some degree or another, could happen in any other EMS system but yours.

Imagine a crew gets the dreaded end-of-shift call—a patient assist who just wants to be picked up off the floor and put back in his chair. The patient denies any complaints, there are no bones sticking through his skin, but vital signs should be taken on every patient; what's the problem with just guesstimating vital signs? It'll save a couple minutes, and if you don't look, you won't find anything that could bog you down into then having to treat the patient, so why not?

So, to the expert medic's eye, the patient looks like a pulse rate of, oh say, 80, a BP of 120/70, and a respiratory rate of 16; sign here and away we go. The patient gets exactly what he asked for, the agency was saved the expense of overtime, the providers get out of work on time, and everybody's happy. Until the oncoming crew gets dispatched right back to the same location an hour later for the same patient, who fell again, this time resulting in a life-altering and possibly life-ending hip fracture.

The new crew, a captive audience for the next twelve hours, has more than enough time to actually check the patient's vital signs, especially now that he is an obviously treatable patient. And lo and behold, they discover a pulse rate of 32. Hooking the patient up to cardiac monitor reveals something unusual looking. There are P waves before most QRS complexes, but every once in a while, the P waves seem to be missing, along with the rest of the cardiac cycle, resulting in an extended period of asystole, typically followed by a ventricular escape beat. Eventually, but belatedly, a P wave does return. This ends up being diagnosed as sinus arrest or sick sinus syndrome, most likely resulting in a temporary decrease in level of consciousness and probably resulting in the falls the patient has been experiencing. The same decreased perfusion that caused these falls may also have affected the patient's sensibility, so that he was not aware that he may have blacked out briefly or suddenly became weak or dizzy. Had the first crew done their job and simply taken a standard set of vital signs, even though they would have gotten home a little late, the patient may have been spared his current serious injury.

Concurrent quality improvement is where the quality coordinator, medical director, or other EMS officers get out into the streets and see what's actually going on in real-time. One mistaken concept is there's little reason to do this, since the providers won't do anything wrong if they know they're being watched. In the study of behavioral science, this is known as the Hawthorne effect. But despite the previously mentioned axiom that people will do a better job if they know they're being watched, every problem in EMS is not so devious. There are many problems or opportunities for improvement in EMS that could be due to the long-term lack of evaluation and correction. Some real-world issues could not be imagined by supervisors or medical directors sitting in the sanctity of their offices. The only way to see what's going on in the streets is to get out into the street.

One such example of this was an observation by coauthor Dr. David Jaslow, the medical director for Bucks County Rescue Squad, that some paramedics were not taking the cardiac monitor into the patient's house unless it was reported to be a cardiac arrest prior to their arrival. Dr. Jaslow observed that the cardiac monitor is the only piece of equipment we carry that can save a patient's life (by virtue of its defibrillator). He argued that a paramedic leaving the monitor in the ambulance was akin to a firefighter leaving his hose line on the engine or a police officer leaving his gun in the patrol car.

Lending credence to Dr. Jaslow's point is the advancements in cardiac monitor capabilities. Older models of cardiac monitors had two lead rhythm monitoring and defibrillation capabilities. Newer generation of monitors are now, for all intents and purposes, complete patient assessment packages, possessing the capability to take and record heart rate, blood pressure, and pulse oximetry—pretty much all the data we would need (minus the actual feeling for a pulse, to do a complete assessment). Some monitors even acquire the respiratory rate through one of the ECG chest leads. Whether you agree with Dr. Jaslow or not, this was an issue that no one would ever have been able to identify by sitting in a room reading PCRs after the fact.

Supervisory quality auditing: There are several ways to do concurrent quality auditing, depending upon your position within the system, your availability, and the flexibility of your system. If you hold an officer's position with supervisory status, you may have the ability to respond to the scene of calls in a supervisor's vehicle. Officers in most systems do this, but it's almost exclusively restricted to large-scale fires, mass casualty incidents (MCIs), or other long-duration incidents such as Hazmats. So what you end up with, with regard to concurrent quality auditing, is the same thing most frequently done with the retrospective review: only high-intensity, high-profile calls are audited.

While MCIs and long-duration incidents clearly do require more on-site management than the single-patient call, supervision, management, and quality auditing should not be exclusively limited to just those types of calls. In the grand scheme of things, MCIs and long-duration incidents represent maybe 5 percent of your call volume, but typically end up getting 100 percent of the supervisory attention, while the remaining 95 percent of your call volume is all but ignored. Regardless of the business your in, any operation that is 95 percent unsupervised is highly likely to have widespread and ongoing problems, especially if this has been a long-standing practice, as is the case with many EMS systems.

Emergent supervisory response is not necessary for quality auditing of single-patient calls. You could leisurely drive to the scene upon dispatch and stop by just to see how things were going. You could even hide this increased supervision in plain sight, by advertising the new policy of increased officer or supervisor "support" on calls. It's a well-known fact that two-person EMS crews are not the most practical for all types of calls. Depending upon your system, your crews may call for an engine company or second unit to assist on cardiac arrests, bariatric (obese) patients, or other difficult calls. Other times or in other systems, the crews may just opt to do the best they can on their own. If your increased involvement is billed as a kinder, gentler supervision, offering your assistance (and even actually lending a hand) when you get there, there's a good chance it will be welcomed with open arms. You should be able to assist with lifting or playing go-fer while at the same time auditing the handling of the call, thus killing two EMS birds with one stone.

Observing and evaluating: Some systems mandate the quality coordinator to ride one shift per year (or certain period of time) with each provider. This is more intrusive and obvious than showing up to offer help and observing the providers in their natural habitat. If a supervisor or quality coordinator is going to ride a shift with a provider, the chances are you're not going to witness totally normal behavior. But as previously mentioned, you will discover many problems that are not malicious or intentional, they're simply the result of poor or inefficient practices that have been perpetuated over the years, due to lack of supervision or clinical feedback. They also may be opportunities for improvement of efficiency or safety that may only be apparent by a neutral observer viewing the big picture.

CHAPTER 8

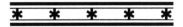

Prospective Quality Improvement

EMS is the front line of emergency medicine and the public safety net.
—Dr. David Jaslow, medical director, Bucks County Rescue Squad

Prospective quality improvement is anything done prior to call dispatch that can improve the quality of care, such as in-service training, continuing education, clinical memoranda, and so on.

Con-ed vs. continuing education: Con-ed is a fact of EMS life. It's the minimum continuing education credits required to maintain active status, with the emphasis on minimum. But who holds a job involving life-and-death decisions and actions on a regularly basis and is satisfied to do only the bare bones minimum? Is that the kind of doctor you'd want to trust your life to? We all get to choose our primary care physician, but no one gets to choose their EMS provider. Patients end up getting whoever happens to be on duty at the time. EMS should be more than just the luck of the draw. We owe it to our patients to always be at our best. At the risk of sounding pretentious, we need to start thinking and acting more like physicians with regard to our commitment to lifelong learning in an attempt to become better emergency medicine providers. EMS is not just a job, it's a profession. People literally place their lives in our hand every day, in reality more so than their family doctors.

Continuing education in some systems has, in many cases, become nothing more than the constant rehashing of the same old canned courses such as Advanced Cardiac Life Support (ACLS). These classes are a great foundation on which to build, but after taking them a couple of times, they mainly end up being more of an update on the latest standards of care than offering any real new educational value.

Call-based education: What has been all but missing from continuing education in EMS is call-based education. Grand rounds come close to this, but just as with retrospective and concurrent quality improvement, they most often end up being relegated to high-profile cases. In addition to that, grand rounds frequently focus on calls with excellent to acceptable management. What would be much more beneficial would be to focus on a call that was poorly managed, especially a type of call that is commonly poorly managed.

One perfect example of this might be how generalized weakness is so frequently underappreciated and undertreated. As previously mentioned, there are many things generalized weakness could be—not all critical emergencies, but many that are, such as stroke, sepsis, cardiac dysrhythmia, MI, and hypoglycemia. Some underlying causes can be confirmed or ruled out in the field by glucometer or EKG, but most cannot. But you don't win points in EMS by guessing right when it's nothing serious, you win points by searching for and finding problems that are not so obvious and erring on the side of caution so you end up ahead of the curve instead of chasing the dragon.

Because the symptom of weakness is so nonspecific, and because in many systems there is not a specific treatment protocol, more often than not the patient is just transported, many times without the provider even checking for the causes they can check for.

You could pull some cases of generalized weakness where the patient ended up being seriously ill. Finding a case where the patient ended up having a bad outcome to dramatize the point would be even better. Putting on a course that focuses on a frequently poorly managed call type identified through the quality improvement process, such as generalized weakness, has the potential to quickly and dramatically improve your standard of care as of the very next shift. That's proactive quality improvement.

The more closely you can link your quality improvement program to your training program, the more quickly you can improve your patient care. Quality improvement and training are the two most important parts of EMS with regard to the actual service we provide, but typically they're two totally separate and distinct entities, which never communicate. For maximum efficiency, the quality improvement and training departments should be partners in marriage with the same goal: improving patient care.

EMS continuing education should not just begin and end with con-ed classes. The quality improvement coordinator is an agent of management. As previously mentioned, while there has typically been excellent supervision in EMS with regard to nonmedical, in-station maintenance tasks, there has traditionally been very little supervision on the medical end of the operation. The time has come for EMS managers to reclaim their role as managers of the actual business of EMS.

Online training: It is a universal, but sometimes forgotten, concept in EMS that employers have the right to dictate how they want their employees to perform the job they're paying them to do. It is perfectly appropriate for an employer or agent of the employer to mandate additional in-house, on-the-clock education. There are many excellent online EMS education sites. In some cases, such as Pennsylvania, the State Department of Health hosts a free online learning management system for use by all certified EMS providers. Despite being available for a few years now, it was only within the last couple of years that the agencies where I coordinate quality improvement have decided to mandate completion of a certain selection of these online courses. It may sound a bit dictatorial to some, but what's so horrible about mandating a half hour of online training to be completed per month, at the employee's convenience, while being paid to do so, on a subject that can help them perform their job better?

In-house library: Every EMS agency has a collection of EMS-related publications lying around on desks, shelves, as well as on the end tables of the duty crew room. Any publications that reference treatment with chloroform and a hack saw or are otherwise outdated should be disposed of. Any still relevant publications should be gathered up and put in a common area.

At a minimum, a current ACLS and PALS provider manual, the most up-to-date treatment protocols for your service, and any additional local, county, or regional operations manuals should be readily available to your providers. While there's no guarantee they'll be read from cover to cover, the availability of such documents dramatically increases the likelihood that providers will know of their existence and possibly even reference them from time to time. Keeping such publications stashed away in an office without universal access defeats the whole purpose of their existence.

Additionally, perhaps the agency could be convinced to purchase some additional reference books and manuals such as Rosen's *Emergency Medicine* or Harrison's *Principal of Internal Medicine*. The idea is not to try and make doctors out of medics but rather encourage them to do call research and learn more about emergency medicine. With the exception of a few manual skills, the more providers know about their discipline of medicine, the better providers they will become. Management has the obligation to assist providers with improving their knowledge. The perfect time to do call research is immediately after a question is encountered on a call. The chances are much greater that providers will do this if reference material is readily available.

Online research: Some books in medicine are available only in standard format, though most are now available electronically and can be downloaded to a PC. There are also many excellent free medical resources available online; www.medlineplus.org has an excellent medical dictionary and encyclopedia, www.drugs.com is very good for quick drug look-up, and www.emedicine.com is an excellent source for emergency medicine literature. To make it more convenient for providers at both our agencies, we added a shortcut/icon for each of these websites on all desktop computers.

Quality improvement newsletter/bulletin: Identify an area in need of improvement, such as the inequity of how various medics treat cardiac chest pain. Write a one-page review of the highlights of the assessment and treatment of ischemic chest pain. Emphasize the importance of early aspirin administration and 12-lead acquisition if applicable to your service. Emphasize the importance of a thoughtful working diagnosis. Not all chest pain is ischemic and therefore should not receive cardiac meds, but all chest pain patients at a minimum should probably receive cardiac monitoring and a 12-lead ECG if available by your agency. Emphasize the importance of standardized care, so that every patient receives the same standard of care no matter which medic they may end up getting.

When writing up a newsletter or bulletin on a patient care topic, you should reference multiple sources and emphasize and reinforce the need for standard of care. Look for and include some interesting and meaningful tidbits of information, such as the fact that early administration of aspirin, chewed for rapid absorption in the AMI patient, has shown a survival rate comparable to that of tPA, the primary clot-busting drug used in ERs for thrombolysis. It is extremely important to keep the newsletter or bulletin topics short, sweet, and to the point—no more than one page, medium to large print, to encourage more providers to actually read it. Use bolding and underlining to emphasis key points so those providers who may not even read one whole page might still walk away learning something just by glancing at it. There's also the hope that if something is bolded or underlined and it grabs the readers' attention, they may actually read the rest of article.

You may also opt to print the newsletter or bulletin on the brightest paper you can find. I used the organizational colors of both squads . . . on steroids. For Bucks County Rescue Squad, this ended up being international orange and electric blue, where the traditional EMS colors of orange and blue were used. At Central Bucks Ambulance, I used lime green and screaming yellow. I alternated colors of the newsletter every other month. If nothing else, this should help draw attention, and that's half the battle with quality improvement.

Lastly, display and distribution is critical. As with every aspect of quality improvement, being imaginative is worth its weight in gold. At one agency, where every provider has a mailbox, I distributed them that way. At the other agency, I scattered a few newsletters around tables and computer stations or anywhere else providers tend to congregate. But my most imaginative and effective measure by far was posting the newsletter over the urinal in the men's room and on the back of the commode door in the ladies' room, taking full advantage of my captive audience and tricking them into learning when they least expected it. I've had several people come up to me and say they learned more going to the potty than they did in some con-ed classes they've taken.

For those providers who will read more than just one page, search the Internet for supportive literature for your newsletter or bulletin topic. You could even highlight the title, and if you really wanted to spoon feed them, highlight the key points in the article. I've done that on occasion. Then leave a copy or two around the station.

Once you get established with the newsletter or bulletin, you should try and invite other providers to contribute to them. If you schmooze them just right, they may be flattered to be asked. The one thing I realized after doing several of these newsletters was that I ended up learning more by researching and writing them. This validates the old adage that the best way to learn something is to teach it. So why not share the wealth? An especially good segue to doing this is tapping the provider who just had an interesting call, or better yet, a provider who had a call in which there were problems.

Quality improvement general announcements: Simple, specific issues that do not require a lot of background information or supportive material, uncovered by the quality improvement process, may be handled by the memo or posted notice method. Likewise, any critical issue that requires immediate action should be printed up and distributed immediately. Some examples of this are when we discovered that medical command was not being called for patient refusal authorization for syncopes, aspirin was being administered inconsistently, or copies of EKGs were not being included with the PCR.

As with the newsletter or bulletin, we choose to use bright paper for attention-getting purposes; one general announcement was placed in each provider's mailbox to ensure all providers were notified. But just to leave nothing to chance, as a last-minute reminder, we additionally posted it on the all doors leading to the apparatus room floor, so it was literally the last thing providers saw before taking a call. As a general rule, no more than three issues (or five or six sentences) should be included in a general announcement. Here is an example:

Quality Improvement
General Announcement

Medical command must be called for *all* patient refusals.

ASA X4 should be administered for all suspected
ischemic chest pain or AMI.

Don't forget to attach a copy of the ECG to the PCR.

Quality corner: At both agencies, I requested and was granted permission to create a quality improvement bulletin board, where the newsletters are posted in addition to any other pertinent materials, such as a manufacturer's poster showing IO administration, 12-lead electrode placement, a sample 12-lead showing the contiguous lead's relationship, and so on.

At the top of the quality improvement bulletin board, I permanently posted one of the ten commandments of quality EMS: "EMS is the first hour of medicine in the first thirty minutes," to stroke the pride of providers and remind them of the extraordinary job they're capable of doing.

Conferences, conventions, and seminars: Another idea for call-based education is to ask the chief to send a few members to any state, regional, or national EMS conferences, conventions, or seminars. This is a target-rich environment that brings the leading experts and best educators and lecturers in EMS together under one roof to present the latest, greatest standards, recommendations, and strategies in EMS today. It's also an environment like the conventions of other professions, which encourages professionalism.

Skills competency verification: EMTs and paramedics complete their initial provider-specific training, along with any clinical preceptorships, and then join the EMS work force. Over the years, technology changes and treatment protocols come and go (hopefully with in-service training being offered to keep providers updated). But with many EMS personnel working multiple jobs, there's always the potential for some providers to miss these updates. Even if you're sure that all present staff have been sufficiently trained on new equipment, new hires after the fact may fall between the cracks. New personnel are typically indoctrinated with a review of the agency's equipment, but some providers may look at a piece of equipment and assume its operation is obvious, say so, and be believed. In addition to providers who fall between the cracks of training, there's also skills degradation. This is especially true for rarely used equipment or procedures, which most typically end up being the most critical interventions.

Several years ago, Dr. Gerry Wydro, medical director of Penndel-Middletown Emergency Squad in Bucks County, recognized the need for and implemented an annual skills competence verification for his agency's providers. Within the last couple of years, Bucks County Rescue Squad, Central Bucks Ambulance, and most other EMS agencies in the county have followed Dr. Wydro's lead.

Despite Dr. Wydro's warning, the first time every agency held skills verification reviews, the results were shocking. Although the majority of providers demonstrated acceptable competency, in every instance there were a few who did not. Some of the more common issues among advanced providers encountered were lack of familiarity operating the transcutaneous pacer, difficulty in setting up and operating CPAP, and failure to hit the "Synch" button for synchronized cardioversion. There were also a couple of instances of inappropriately placed needles for pleural decompressions. Needless to say, all these issues were quickly fixed, but these were problems no medical director or quality coordinator could have imagined existed.

The moral of this lesson was until and unless proficiency is actually verified, do not make the mistake of assuming it's always being performed appropriately. Any issues with patient care left unidentified and unresolved have the potential for disaster. Rarely used critical interventions are the best place to start looking for such issues.

CHAPTER 9

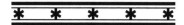

Managing Your Quality Program

One of the secrets to life is learning how to make stepping stones out of stumbling blocks.
—Jack Penn

Don't forget the good: Despite the primary objective of quality improvement being to identify and correct problems in the pursuit of improved patient care, a progressive quality program should not be all negative. On any given day, there are more things going right in EMS than wrong. This should be emphasized at every opportunity and in every way so the program is as encouraging as it is educational. Good quality coordinators not only identify and correct problems, they also look for opportunities to acknowledge excellence.

Letters of commendation: Compliments are the gold medal of quality improvement. One day perhaps we'll have a real gold medal to give, but for right now, compliments will have to do. When providers have, in the view of the peer quality reviewer or medical director, done an exceptionally good job or handled a difficult call well, they should be recognized, and a letter of commendation is an easy and affordable way of doing so. The original should be given to the provider and a copy should be placed in the provider's QI file.

Awards: Every time I walk into the Bucks County Rescue Squad, I pass a trophy case full of awards that go back to 1932. Over the years, as volunteer rescue squads and ambulance corps in Pennsylvania gave way to the paid EMS agencies of today, banquets and annual awards have fallen by the wayside. That's unfortunate, because for anyone who didn't know better, seeing all those awards from yesteryear and nothing from today, they'd have to wonder what's wrong with these underachievers today or be left to ask, so what have you done lately? Since we're doing more and better things than ever before in EMS, why shouldn't we acknowledge that fact in ways that positively reinforce the kind of behavior we're seeking, as well as showcase those achievements on behalf of the agency?

As a result of this awareness, we commissioned three awards: the Code Buster Award, the Stork Club, and the Top Gun Award. The Code Buster Award is a plaque that acknowledges successful resuscitations. The Stork Club is for baby deliveries in the field. And the last award is one that ended up spurring a surprising amount of competition among providers. The Top Gun Award is for excellence in call management. Just like in the movie, the Top Gun is not an individual award, but rather for an EMS crew or team, which further encourages the team concept.

Within the first six months of the commissioning of those plaques, we had three babies delivered and five successful resuscitations. This was a surprising number of achievements to everyone, but it underscores the fact that you don't realize how much good you're doing in EMS until you take a step back and look. Although not our original intent, these awards helped us do that.

Initially, I envisioned Top Gun being a monthly award. However, our medical director, Dr. David Jaslow, who is both the greatest champion and toughest critic of EMS, insisted upon maintaining the highest standards for the Top Gun award. Consequently, we ended up with seven Top Gun recipients in the first twelve months. Surprisingly, Top Gun ended up being a very competitive, sought-after award by providers.

All three of these awards are large plaques that hang on the wall opposite the main entrance, so they are the first thing anyone sees upon entering the building.

The one-third rule: Typically, about one third of EMS providers will do a good job with little or no supervision; another one third will do a good job when asked, encouraged, or coached to; and the last third will only do a good job if they're counseled, ordered, or threatened to do so under penalty of termination. Ultimately, the more providers you can recruit for employment in the top two categories, the better. But as with most systems, you're inevitably going to be saddled with some of the lower third echelon who, for various personal reasons, will challenge and resist you every step of the way.

Quality improvement is a confidential process: Like HIPAA, any quality issues are strictly confidential. No member of the quality improvement team should ever discuss any QI-related issues with anyone other than those persons directly affected by the issue. Additionally, confidentiality should be required of any other parties who may have to be interviewed or involved in the process.

There is no one in EMS or any practice of medicine who has not and will not make an error, including the medical director and quality coordinator. Because no one is exempt from errors, no provider should be exempt from the quality improvement process, including the quality coordinator (if they are still an active practitioner). Publicizing this fact should earn some degree of respect and feeling of fairness, if not enthusiasm. The objective of quality improvement is to identify and correct errors and provide educational feedback to the provider, it is not to embarrass them or damage their reputation.

Trends: If a poor or questionable practice is identified by multiple providers, it's typically considered a trend. The need for correction of a trend is just as important as, if not more important than, an individual issue depending on the practice in question, because it is mass produced. Corrective action of a trend can be executed by an all-hands meeting if possible or correspondence to all providers. Additionally, a notice should be posted briefly explaining the problem and corrective action. The more modes and times that a concept is repeated, the more likely and quickly a change in behavior can be expected. So, if a quick and critical change in behavior is required, consider a multiprong attack of the problem: memos to all providers and posting a notice.

Letters of inquiry: For questionable calls and even many poorly managed calls, a letter of inquiry sent to the provider may allow for clarification. There are a couple of reasons for this. First, it permits the provider to explain his or her logic. One of the most common problems in EMS has always been (and probably will continue to be) documentation, most notably omissions. But even more importantly, we found that the discomfort associated with having to answer an official inquiry makes it far less likely the provider will repeat the action or inaction in the future. Any constructive criticism or inquiry of action will typically be much better received if coming from the higher medical authority (such as the medical director) rather than a peer provider. Ideally, medical directors should sign any such correspondence or have their name appear as the initiator. Adding his credentials to any official correspondence is also appropriate; for example, Ben Casey, MD, MPH, FAAEM.

Corrective action letter: Cases of a clearly poorly managed call, inappropriate deviations from protocols, or poor clinical judgment should be pointed out respectfully. An explanation of why the action or inaction in question was inappropriate and how a more appropriate action or treatment option would have been better should be included. A corrective action letter might be even more effective if medical literature supporting the correction is included.

One example of this might be where a patient was in severe respiratory distress and the working diagnosis was CHF, but CPAP was not utilized. Along with the corrective action letter, a copy of an article explaining the mechanics and efficacy of CPAP could be included.

With the Internet and all the excellent search engines such as Google at your disposal, there is no shortage of medical literature that can quickly and easily be accessed, printed off, and sent to providers. A couple of the best free resources I've found for this are www.emedicine.com and www. medlineplus.org.

Casual counseling: In lieu of a letter of inquiry or corrective action letter, if the provider in question is readily available, the quality coordinator (or ideally the medical director) may opt to casually counsel the provider regarding an issue. Dr. Jaslow does this whenever possible, since it's more personal and less intimidating than receiving official correspondence. It also allows for personal interaction, since you can't ask a letter a question. But even more importantly, it shows active involvement and interest on the part of the medical director; consequently, the medical director may no longer be seen as the unapproachable man or woman behind the curtain.

Official counseling and remediation: Most quality issues can be resolved by correspondence or casual counseling. Occasionally, when a major concept in emergency medicine management seems to have been missed or in cases of repeated mismanagement, educational remediation may be necessary. If a provider does not seem to have a firm grasp on the current standards of emergency cardiac care, the medical director might consider mandating the provider to retake an ACLS course. If a provider demonstrates a deficiency in intubations, the medical director may mandate the provider perform intubations in the OR or ER. The medical director may also opt to personally counsel a provider regarding any specific issue of concern. In cases where more than one attempt at correcting a problem via correspondence has failed, a counseling session with the medical director should be mandated. Letters and e-mails are easy to ignore; refusing to heed the advice or orders of the medical director, face to face, is not so easy. Overtly ignore the physician under whose license you practice, and you may no longer be practicing. One concept that is universally understood in all the rest of medicine, but not always in EMS, is that any practice of medicine is a privilege awarded to doctors by hospitals or other health care institutions, and in the case of paramedics, permitted at the EMS agency by the medical director. If at any time the medical director loses confidence in the EMS provider to perform prehospital emergency medical care safely and competently, they could and should revoke their medical command privilege.

M&M conferences: You've seen it on TV's *E.R.* and other medical shows. An intern screws up and the patient dies or has a bad outcome. The next day, the errant doctor is standing in front of a panel of senior physicians, and typically with an entire audience of their peers, sweating bullets as they present their case, point out the errors they made, and answer some very tough questions fired at them from the panel. M&M, or morbidity and mortality, conferences are a common training tool throughout medicine, but typically unheard of in EMS. But perhaps the time has come to start treating paramedics like the grown-up health care providers we want them to be. The reason M&M conferences are so effective is because they are so painful; once you go through one of them, you never want to go through another and are therefore very unlikely to repeat the same mistake.

Peer pressure: Posting individual provider statistics (e.g., paramedics' ALS treatment rates and patient refusal rates) by certification number can be a very effective way to get peer pressure working for you. We did this at one agency after not being pleased with the pace of our progress. This was the chief's idea. Originally I didn't think it was a good idea, but you can't argue with success. No one wants to see their name or number at the bottom of any list for fear of everyone finding out who they are. Surprisingly to me, the treatment statistics started moving up quickly after that.

Quality files: First and foremost, quality improvement files are detailed proof that you truly have a quality improvement program. While the existence of quality improvement files may not be too important today, when the time comes, sometime in the future, for some sort of comprehensive audit of EMS—and it will—you'll be ready. This is another example of where you can choose to stay ahead of the curve now or play catch-up later.

Every provider should have a quality improvement file. For some providers, the mere knowledge of the existence of such a file could be a deterrent to problems, along the lines of how the dreaded "permanent record" in elementary school kept so many students in line. Probably not the most flattering example of motivation within EMS, but the reality is, you will be dealing with a wide range of personalities, and different techniques will work for different personality types.

Provider quality improvement files should contain letters of commendation, letters of inquiry, as well as the provider's responses to any inquiries, corrective action letters and complaints, and any other pertinent documentation related to their quality of care.

Provider quality improvement files also become critically important in cases where quality issues must be raised to the level of disciplinary action, such as repetitive issues or where the provider simply refuses to cooperate with the quality improvement process.

Provider quality improvement files may also alert you to a trend, which could indicate that a provider may not have the proper temperament to be an EMS provider. What has all but gone unmentioned in EMS is the fact that this is not a job just anyone can do. It is possible that someone could complete all the didactic and clinical requirements but simply not be capable of functioning to an acceptable level of competency in the real world of EMS.

We in EMS are frequently called upon to operate in the most critical, austere, and difficult situations. Pressure is a variable they do not and cannot totally test for in the classroom. But pressure is the wild card of variables in the practice of paramedicine. Pressure will cause some people to focus and others to crack. Needless to say, this could be a difficult situation to handle, but like anything else with regard to QI issues, it's probably best to know it exists, rather than find out as a result of tragedy (or worse yet, repeated tragedies). Having documentation that paints a comprehensive picture to make your case is much more effective than just having a hunch, suspicion, or innuendo, no matter how right you may be.

Probation/termination: As has been stated many times, quality improvement should be primarily educational, not punitive. However, there are exceptions to every rule, and quality improvement in EMS is no exception. The instances requiring discipline in quality improvement should be rare, but when all else fails, you cannot shy away from doing what has to be done to ensure patient safety. EMS is not just a job, it is a profession, and it's about time it started being treated like it. Patients place their lives in our hands every day. If you cannot control or trust a provider, you must not shrink away from the task, unpleasant though it may be, of getting rid of them.

If a provider repeatedly deviates from protocols or the standard of care of your agency or refuses to cooperate with the quality improvement process, you may opt to either put them on probation or terminate them, depending upon the severity of the infraction. This will most likely be a judgment call.

Some subset of problem providers, like employees anywhere else, simply will not be willing to modify their behavior no matter what, believing that they are right and the entire rest of the system is wrong. In these cases, when reasonable attempts at correcting the problem have failed, it may be necessary to terminate the provider. If the issue is more operational in nature, such as attitudinal by refusing to cooperate with the process, you may want to lay a carrot and a stick on the table; for example, give them the option of resigning to maintain a clean record rather than be fired. A word of caution here, be extremely careful when using the carrot-and-stick approach. If the provider is a true danger to patient care, you should avoid using this method. It is morally wrong to push a dangerous provider someplace else to continue their hazardous practice without giving others fair warning. Part of the purpose of official sanctions, such as medical command being withdrawn or restricted, is to document such issues. If the provider should go on to harm a patient, the case ends up in the courts, and it comes to light that you discovered the problem but did not document or report it in accordance with state or regional guidelines, you could be held liable. It is important to know the quality improvement guidelines and responsibilities for your region and state.

No one enjoys firing someone and being a party to them losing their livelihood and turning their life upside down. But you can't shy away from doing what needs to be done when it comes to patient safety. Also, keep in mind it is the noncompliant employee who is ultimately responsible for his or her own fate, not you. It is also reasonable and logical to assume that if a person loses his or her job, whether due to performance, attendance, or whatever, he or she would be forced to confront the problem and hopefully make the necessary changes or risk a repeat of the very unpleasant experience.

Short of termination, there is probation. Probation may be administrative or clinical probation, depending upon whether management or the medical director takes the lead. As a matter of fairness, probation should not be open-ended (that is, last indefinitely), notwithstanding the legal ramifications. A reasonable probation period should be no less than ninety days and no more than six months, depending on the severity of the issue.

If any additional significant issues develop with that provider within the prescribed probationary time, you are in an excellent position to terminate the provider. Termination, however, is most likely an action that will have to be executed by management on your recommendation. Consequently, as soon as termination is considered, whether immediately or as a possible outcome of a probationary period, management needs to be advised and involved.

Confidential sources have proven to be a valuable resource for me. Most EMS providers are conscientious. They know when another provider is taking short cuts and usually are not totally comfortable with it. But prior to a real quality improvement program being established, they typically had no recourse. In many cases, they may be the junior member of the crew, such as an EMT working with a medic. Despite the paramedic many times having six whole months to a year more training than the EMT, in most agencies, the medic will be given the benefit of the doubt in any controversy, sometimes even if it's felt the EMT was technically correct.

Reason being, the dogma attached to questioning a higher medical authority. I personally know of more than one conscientious EMT who has been fired over this. Even if you are right, if this is your livelihood, you can't afford to be right too many times.

Barring an extraordinary situation that demands immediate and drastic action, you should protect and preserve your confidential sources. Even in critical situations that may require quick action, consider using your confidential source as an anonymous whistleblower or use the information they've provided to help set up the official identification of the problem that does not implicate the source, such as saying you yourself discovered or stumbled onto the problem. As long as the factual details are presented, it will be difficult to refute.

Understand that your responsibility to protect confidential sources is a moral responsibility, which can affect the Good Samaritan's career and livelihood. If the incident is so egregious that maintaining confidentiality is not possible, you may first want to go to management to make your case. Without mentioning the name of the source, make them aware of the magnitude of the problem and point out how much they owe the source for uncovering it. Emphasize the risk of the problem not being dealt with and make sure they see this person as a hero with the best interest of the patient and the agency in mind. Try to get an assurance of the source's job security, then advise your source of the situation before any action is taken. Like a newspaper reporter, if you want to maintain a source, you must protect the source. Betray them just once and you'll have lost that source forever, as well as other potential sources once word gets out.

None of us are as smart as all of us: One major problem that has held EMS back and made all of our jobs more difficult for so long is the fact that we have not always communicated well or been willing to share our knowledge with each other. Considering the limited resources of much of EMS, it's ridiculous that every agency must find the same solution to so many of the same problems. Once a solution to a problem or better way of doing something is discovered, it should be shared if at all possible. If, on the other hand, the concept of a successful initiative is offered, you should not reject or ignore it simply because it was not your original idea. This mentality has for far too long caused unnecessary duplication of effort, wasted time, and delay in improving patient care. Quality improvement in EMS is not a zero-sum game, as is the case in elections and wrestling matches, where someone must lose in order for someone to win.

If all surrounding agencies were to raise their standard of care based on your initiative, it does not detract from your success; rather it magnifies it—exponentially. It is also an achievement for which you should take great pride. Notwithstanding, the life saved in the next district due to you sharing what you've learned could well end up being someone you know.

Conversely, if you know of a colleague who has achieved success with her quality improvement program, you should seek them out and inquire how they did it. Most people would find it flattering to be asked for their wise advice and counsel, especially if expressed in that manner.

If adapted, you should always acknowledge and give full credit to the originator of any borrowed initiative. To do so makes you look classy, and truth be told, it really does not distract much at all from the perception of you as a leader, because in the final analysis, successful managing is not about doing everything yourself, it's about seeking out, recruiting, and implementing the best ideas that can be found from any source. The chief of operations or board of directors will not care one bit if you were to dramatically improve your agency's patient care by implementing an initiative borrowed from somewhere else, and neither will your patients, rather they will be every bit as grateful as if it were your original idea.

Since all of us in EMS share so many of the same problems, the time has come to start organizing, networking, and working smarter, not harder, to improve our patient care. Leading this effort is *EMS World* magazine, which in January 2011 commissioned the *Quality Corner* webpage. This column is hosted by the author of this book, Joe Hayes, and Dr. Ken Lavelle, the medical director for Central Bucks Ambulance. In breaking convention with most columns, the hosts of the column encourage quality coordinators from across the country to share their ideas and thoughts on quality improvement by contributing as guest columnists, because none of us are as smart as all of us.

CHAPTER 10

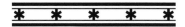

Tracking Your Progress
Statistics and In-House Studies

An error is not a mistake until you fail to correct it.
—Anonymous

Statistics—use with caution: Robert McNamara was the secretary of defense under Presidents Kennedy and Johnson. But before that, he was a systems analyst for the Army Air Corp during World War II. It was in this capacity that he demonstrated the value of using statistics in war. He convinced General Curtis LeMay that the number of bombers aborting their mission before reaching their targets due to mechanical failures was statistically improbable. The other obvious possibility—pilots were aborting their missions because they were afraid of being killed.

Armed with this information, General LeMay addressed his troops, advising them of their suspicion and a new policy. First of all, from that moment on, he would fly the lead plane on all bombing missions, and secondly, anyone who turned back and was found not to have a mechanical problem would be court-martialed. Aborted bombing missions immediately fell to near zero. Robert McNamara was exalted as a statistical genius and given a medal.

Beyond the statistics and suspicions of McNamara, what has never been made clear is whether he guessed right or actually went to talk to the mechanics to verify what he thought his statistics were telling him. There is such a thing as manufacturer's defect, after all. But either way, he was proven to be correct in this case.

Fast forward to the 1960s; Robert McNamara is secretary of defense and dubbed the architect of the Vietnam War. Like old generals who always refight their last great battle, McNamara immediately employed the tool that worked so well for him in World War II, only now he attempts to manage an entire war based on statistics, such as tonnage of bombs dropped and body counts. In this case, we now know those statistics were never correlated with reality. The victory in the making they repeatedly assured the American people of was prejudiced by what they wanted to see instead of verified by the facts on the ground. The end result, of course, was the complete opposite of what was believed.

Statistics are a valuable management tool, if used properly. We use them in the quality improvement program at both Bucks County Rescue Squad and Central Bucks Ambulance. In addition to our two little EMS agencies, statistics are what drive all the rest of medicine in what has come to be known as evidenced-based medicine. Statistics are a measurement tool; they can demonstrate constants or change, but they cannot tell you what the underlying causes of those trends are. To give any meaning to statistics, you must always correlate what you think they mean with the actual detail data.

You don't need to be a mathematician to crunch meaningful statistics for the purposes of quality improvement. The math is simple: addition and division. The math is made simpler still if you use a calculator, which all PCs have under the Accessory programs. There are many ways of measuring progress, but for the purpose of some quick and easy statistics to monitor your progress, here's what we did.

Number of calls: First we recorded our total number of patient/calls per month. Notice I did not just say calls. One call could have more than one patient. There could also be no patient found on a call. We basically counted the number of PCRs generated and titled it "Patient/Calls." You can track the number of dispatched calls, the number of patient contacts, or whatever you prefer. All that matters is that you calculate it the same way every time, otherwise you end comparing apples to oranges. So for September 2009, the Bucks County Rescue Squad had 329 patient/calls or PCRs generated. We typically compare the number of patient/calls for the present month with the number of patient/calls from the same month of the previous year to see if our call volume was decreasing or increasing. In most cases, they increased. Surprisingly, as a dramatic departure from our pretty consistently increasing call volume, we discovered during the recession that our call volume decreased slightly over several months, possibly due to the financial concerns of people.

Number of patient refusals: Depending on the PCR system you have, patient refusals may have subcategories. We use the Pinpoint PCR system by Zoll. In Pinpoint, there are subcategories such as "Refusal Treatment," "Refusal Treatment and Transport," and "Treatment No Transport." You may also want to look at other non-transport categories, such as "Call Cancelled" and "Recalled." Many EMS providers probably believe there's more oversight going on than there actually is, so some of the more laid back providers may try and hide patient refusals in other less indicting categories. Again the most important thing is however you calculate it, do it the same way every time.

A word of caution here regarding refusals: 10 percent is a frequently suggested average, but one bus accident or other mass casualty incident with no injuries or several minor injuries could obviously skew that number. A jump in any statistic you're using to monitor patient care will quickly alert you to a change in the norm, but you should never assume anything positive or negative based upon just that number alone. It should only alert you to the need to take a closer look at the underlying detail data to try and identify the cause.

One modification we eventually decided to implement with our patient refusal rate at Bucks County Rescue Squad was to report multiple refusals from a single incident, most typically motor vehicle crashes as a single refusal. The reason being, we didn't want the number to look worse because a diligent provider got a refusal for everyone involved, which is optimal, versus a lower number of refusals where a provider chose to get just a single patient refusal for an incident despite multiple persons being involved. Again, you can tweak these statistics any way that makes sense to you, but if you're going to be using them as a measurement tool, you want to use the same yardstick every time.

ALS treatment rate: Another category we look at monthly is the ALS treatment rate. We calculate this by dividing the number of ALS treatments by the total number of patient treatments, that is, total ALS and BLS treatments. If your agency runs BLS as well as ALS ambulances, for purposes of calculating the ALS treatment rate, you should only count the number of BLS treatments by the ALS unit. In other words, do not count the BLS treatments by BLS units, since ALS treatment is not an option for them even if it is warranted. What you're looking for here is the ratio of ALS to BLS treatments by your medic units. In addition to the ALS vs. BLS treatment ratio, you will probably want to report the total number of BLS treatments by all type units—ALS and BLS.

Again be cognizant of your PCR system's categories. In addition to the obvious category of ALS Treatment, there could be additional qualifying subcategories. Once again using the Pinpoint model as an example, there are such subcategories as ALS Treatment on BLS (transporting) Unit and Care Transferred to another service, such as Medevac.

Legitimate treatment and releases should also be counted. An example of this might be the hypoglycemic diabetic who is treated with IV dextrose, has thier blood sugar and mental status restored, and then refuses transport with appropriate discharge instructions and medical command authorization. I've also recently begun to notice a trend of some minor asthma attacks being given a breathing treatment and then refusing transport with medical command authorization. As insurance companies become more aware of the financial savings with field treatments instead of full ER visits for certain appropriate cases, we could see the number of treat and releases increase.

It's up to you to determine what your optimum ALS treatment rate should be. The goal is not to just blindly strive for a number just for the numbers' sake, but if you're paying medics more money than EMTs to provide ALS care and they're failing to treat a significant number of patients who should or could benefit by ALS, then your agency is probably not getting what they're paying for. As an agent of the employer, you have the authority in conjunction with the medical director to set the standard of care and insist that it be met. As previously mentioned, this authority has been abdicated by many agencies and totally left to the discretion of each and every individual provider, which is as dangerous as it is ridiculous.

Total patient treatments: A monthly total of patient treatments may also be kept. This is the sum of both ALS and BLS treated patients. This should include treat and releases and transfer of care, since they are legitimate treatments.

At a minimum, you should check the above statistics each month. If you compare these numbers against the baseline statistics before you began your quality improvement program, you should see significant (and hopefully consistent) improvement over time. The difference in the before and after statistics is one way to prove your quality improvement program is having an impact.

Other in-house studies: Looking at and improving patient refusal and ALS treatment rates is a good place to start and a foundation on which to build, but they do not tell you about the efficacy of care. For that, you'll have to look a little deeper.

The first efficacy of treatment indicator we decided to look at was chest pains. We identified the total number of chest pain calls for a three-month period. We then counted the number of those patients who received 12-lead ECGs, aspirin, nitroglycerine, and morphine. For accuracy, you'll first need to identify and split the chest pain calls into the two main working diagnostic categories of suspected ischemic and non-ischemic chest pain. This is important since it would be inappropriate to treat non-ischemic chest pain with anything other than possibly an ECG.

Chest Pain	Ischemic	Non Ischemic	ECG	ASA	NTG	MSO_4
25	19	6	20/80%	12/63%	13/68%	4/ 21%

Statistical formulas shown below

20 ECGs / 25 total chest pains = 80%
12 aspirin admin. / 19 Ischemic chest pains = 63% ASA adm. ischemic chest pain
13 nitroglycerine adm. / 19 ischemic chest pains = 68%
4 morphine adm. / 19 ischemic chest pains = 21%

The American Heart Association has determined that early 12-lead ECG and aspirin administration are the top two priorities for any suspected acute coronary syndrome patient. Based on that, these numbers looked like they could use some improvement. The quality improvement coordinator, along with the medical director, should determine whether the rest of these numbers are acceptable. Either way, just as with the refusal and ALS treatment rates, you now have a quantitative snapshot as far as what your providers are actually doing out there.

If you determine that there is a need for improvement, as we did at both Bucks County Rescue Squad and Central Bucks Ambulance, you could write up a quality improvement newsletter explaining what the expected standard of care is for chest pain. We also posted a notice on all the doors leading to the apparatus room reminding providers to perform 12-lead ECGs on all chest pain or suspected cardiac patients, as well as the importance of early administration of aspirin and attempts to eradicate chest pain believed to be ischemic by nitroglycerine administered up to three times followed by 2 to 5 mg of morphine. We took another look at these same statistics one month later and noticed significant improvement across the board, proof that we could in fact quickly and dramatically improve the quality of our patient care.

Other ad-hoc studies we ran included airway management and efficacy of Versed for facilitated intubation. With regard to airway management, we discovered that our intubation success rate, while not horrible, did leave some room for improvement, so we put on an airway management class.

At one agency, what we discovered by this study, which was even more significant, was the fact that in most cases of failed intubation, the providers were reverting back to BLS airway management instead of employing our rescue airway, which was at the time the Combitube. The reason became immediately apparent to us: it was because of space constraints with our first-in bags. There was no room to store the Combitube with the intubation kits. It was therefore out-of-sight, out-of-mind. Ultimately, we decided to purchase bigger first-in bags so we had room to store the Combitube with the other airway adjuncts. But most immediately, even though knowing the answer, we sent letters of inquiry to all providers who did not use the Combitue for a failed intubation, asking why it was not used. The fact that they had to answer an official inquiry quickly overcame the out-of-sight, out-of-mind issue. None of the providers failed to revert to the Combitube following failed intubations after that, and that's ultimately what we were shooting for. In addition to the letters of inquiry, we also posted a general announcement reminding providers to revert to the Combitube in cases of failed intubation or document why they did not. Within one month, the problem was 100 percent resolved. The only exceptions were two cases where there was continued jaw clenching; the Combitube could therefore not be passed, and that fact was documented in both cases.

For half a dozen years, Versed was the medication assigned to us in Bucks County for facilitated intubation. There were constant complaints among providers of it not working. But anecdotal complaints don't carry much weight in medicine. If you magically save a life by a new or different technique, where you're sure the patient otherwise would have died, and you go to the AMA in hopes of sharing your miracle with the rest of the world, they'll tell you to go back, do a study, and prove it first. Reason being, there are an infinite number of variables besides the one you believe made the difference, including just dumb luck. So before all of medicine adapts your method or treatment, you will first have to prove its efficacy.

With complaints of Versed abounding, we decided to take the groundbreaking step of doing a simple in-house study on the efficacy of Versed for facilitated intubtations. We discovered, in this case, the anecdotal complaints were justified. Versed had a 48 percent success rate for facilitated intubations at one agency and exactly 50 percent at the other. Not a very impressive track record with regard to efficacy of a medication, especially when you consider this was the one typically employed in life-and-death cases of emergency airway management.

One caveat to this Versed saga worth noting came as a result of a concurrent quality audit I did while riding along with providers. I witnessed one difficult airway management case with an unconscious, hypoxic patient with jaw clenching. They appropriately opted to do a facilitated intubation. In the process, I noticed that the one provider pushed the Versed, while the other provider almost immediately went for the intubation. There's no telling if this practice was typical among all providers in our agency, but in this case it was apparent that the Versed was not given sufficient time to take effect prior to the intubation attempt. Despite the reeducation of our providers on the proper technique for facilitated intubation, subsequent statistical studies failed to show any significant improvement in the efficacy of Versed for facilitated intubation. But as we've stated, it's amazing what you can see if you care to look.

EPILOGUE

EMS is the most intense, challenging, and high-stakes practice of medicine there is—bar none. Unlike hospital-based health care, EMS providers operate in an uncontrolled and frequently dangerous environment, without the safety net of specialty resources and back-up. But even at this late date and time in history, in many cases it is still being left up to each and every individual provider to decide what their agency's standard of care should be, which by definition is not a standard of care. When you consider there is more supervision for the people flipping burgers at fast-food restaurants than in many EMS systems, you realize how much work there is to do.

Supervision with regard to the most critical part of EMS—patient care—is still frequently nonexistent in many systems. The fact that the core business of EMS begins when the alerting system activates and the crew leaves the station (and all supervision) behind admittedly presents a unique management challenge, but not an impossible one.

The retrospective review of patient care reports (PCRs) should not just be limited to high-intensive, high-profile calls, which is a popular tendency throughout EMS. Most of the problems with patient care involve routine calls such as generalized weakness, abdominal pains, falls, and patient assists. These are perceived as the boring, unglamorous calls of EMS. Consequently, they're not always taken seriously and properly assessed, and therefore frequently go untreated.

Perhaps most important for ensuring quality patient care is the need for concurrent or real-time quality auditing. Supervisors, quality coordinators, and ideally medical directors need to get out of their offices and into the street, where the real life-and-death work of EMS takes place. Similar to the common error with retrospective quality reviews, the concurrent quality audit process should not be limited to just high-intensity, high-profile calls, such as mass casualty incidents, auto extrications, and large structure fires. Supervisors, quality coordinators, and medical directors need to see how their providers are handling routine calls. Then when EMS providers, in their honest but erroneous opinion, opt to give an elderly patient complaining of acute generalized weakness a "taxi ride" to the hospital without ever attempting to look for an underlying cause, or pick up a fall victim and plop him back into his chair without considering the differential diagnosis, the perfect teaching moment can be seized upon and a major weakness in EMS corrected.

Advanced life support in EMS is physician-level medicine, albeit more focused and restricted. Any paramedic who is trusted to practice this level of medicine with just twelve to twenty-four months of training (compared to the physician's twelve years) must understand and appreciate the incredible trust being bestowed upon them. All EMS providers should never forget that their patients are entrusting their lives to them on every call. Additionally, all emergency medicine practitioners must understand that while people have the luxury of choosing their primary care physician, no one gets to choose their emergency care provider. It is therefore a moral imperative that anyone choosing to practice paramedicine never be satisfied with simply meeting some minimal standard. Like physicians who set the high standard before us, all practitioners of prehospital emergency medicine should be committed to lifelong learning and a deliberate effort to always be at their best for the sake of their patients.

Lastly, EMS education needs to get beyond just the constant rehashing of Advanced Cardiac Life Support and a few other canned courses. High-performance EMS requires the development of call-based education, which is married to deficits in knowledge identified by the quality improvement process. This education is designed to turn technicians who mindlessly administer Albuterol anytime they hear a wheeze into clinicians who better understand the pathophysiology and risk of giving Albuterol to the congestive heart failure patient, who may also present with wheezes.

After thirty years of modern EMS, the time has come to recognize that quality improvement is the core business of EMS and needs to be made the priority it should be, if not because it's the right thing to do, then for self-preservation. The astute observer need only look to the hospitals to realize that stricter compliance of quality patient care will soon be mandated for EMS, not only by law, but by financial reimbursement.